Neuroregeneration and Novel Insights in BORDERLINE EMOTIONAL DISORDERS in Regenerative Medicine

Neuroregeneration and Novel Insights in BORDERLINE EMOTIONAL DISORDERS in Regenerative Medicine

MIKE K. S. CHAN

DINA TULINA

EUROPEAN™ WELLNESS ACADEMY

Biological Regenerative Medicine

Neuroregeneration and Novel Insights in Borderline Emotional Disorders in Regenerative Medicine

EUROPEAN WELLNESS ACADEMY

Library of Congress Control Number: 2026935260

ISBN (hardcover): 9781662971044
eISBN: 9781662972843

DOI: https://doi.org/10.69669/kb2904

gatekeeper press™

Tampa, Florida

Contents

EDUCATIONAL DISCLAIMER

Educational Purpose Only

The information contained in this book is intended solely for educational and informational purposes. This publication serves as educational commentary and analysis of medical topics and should not be construed as professional medical advice, diagnosis, or treatment recommendations. The content is designed to increase health awareness, promote understanding of medical concepts, and support informed decision-making for health matters.

Not a Substitute for Professional Medical Care

The content presented herein is **not intended to replace** consultation with qualified healthcare professionals. Readers should not use the information in this book to diagnose, treat, cure, or prevent any medical condition or disease without first consulting with a licensed physician or other qualified healthcare provider.

Public Education Focus

This educational commentary is intended to:

- Help the general public understand health concepts and terminology
- Provide accessible information about medical topics
- Support general health literacy and awareness
- Promote informed discussions about health matters
- Encourage readers to become more knowledgeable about health topics

Individual Medical Circumstances

Medical conditions, treatments, and responses vary significantly among individuals. What may be appropriate for one person may not be suitable for another. The authors and publishers recognize that each reader's medical situation is unique and requires personalized professional evaluation.

No Doctor-Patient Relationship

Reading this book does not establish a doctor-patient relationship between the reader and the authors, contributors, or publishers. The information provided is general in nature and cannot address specific individual medical circumstances.

Consult Healthcare Professionals

Before making any decisions regarding your health, medical treatment, or medication:

- Consult with your primary care physician
- Seek advice from appropriate medical specialists
- Discuss any questions or concerns with qualified healthcare providers
- Follow the guidance of licensed medical professionals who can evaluate your specific situation

Limitation of Liability

The authors, editors, contributors, and publishers of this book disclaim any liability, loss, injury, or damage incurred as a consequence, directly or indirectly, of the use and application of any of the contents of this publication. This includes, but is not limited to, any adverse reactions, injuries, or health complications that may result from following any suggestions, procedures, or information contained in this book.

Evolving Medical Knowledge

While every effort has been made to ensure the accuracy of the information presented, medical knowledge is constantly evolving. The authors and publishers cannot guarantee that all information is current, complete, or applicable to all situations. Medical standards, treatments, and recommendations may change over time.

Professional Responsibility

Healthcare decisions should always be made in consultation with qualified medical professionals who can:

- Evaluate your complete medical history
- Perform appropriate examinations
- Consider your individual risk factors
- Provide personalized treatment recommendations
- Monitor your progress and adjust treatments as needed

Final Advisory

By reading this book, you acknowledge that you understand and agree to this disclaimer. The authors and publishers are not responsible for any consequences resulting from the use of this educational information. You assume full responsibility for any decisions you make regarding your health and medical care, and you agree to consult with appropriate healthcare professionals before taking any action based on information contained in this publication.

This disclaimer is effective as of the publication date and may be updated periodically. Readers are encouraged to review this disclaimer regularly.

Chapter 1

Borderline disorders: concept and contemporary relevance

"Borderline" mental disorders occupy a clinical and conceptual zone between normal adaptive responses and established psychiatric disease. The term as used here does not refer narrowly to borderline personality disorder, but broadly to subthreshold or early-stage conditions in which individuals experience persistent or recurrent disturbances of mood, stress-responsivity, and anxiety that do not fully meet criteria for major depressive disorder, generalized anxiety disorder, or other categorical diagnoses. These states are characterized by fluctuating symptoms, vulnerability to psychosocial stressors, impaired coping, and a heightened risk of progression to more severe, chronic, or comorbid psychiatric and somatic conditions.

Conceptually, borderline disorders are best understood through a dimensional lens: symptom severity, duration, and functional impact exist along continua rather than as discrete categories. Many affected people present with a mix of sleep disturbance, irritability, low mood, fatigue, cognitive fog, somatic complaints, hypervigilance, and intermittent panic or worry. These symptoms are often temporally linked to psychosocial stressors (job loss, relationship disruption, chronic caregiving, social isolation) but are also shaped by biological vulnerability—genetic predisposition, early-life adversity, metabolic and inflammatory states, and disrupted neurobiological circuits for stress regulation. Because borderline disorders sit between wellness and illness, they are frequently discounted by sufferers and clinicians alike, leading to under-recognition and under-treatment. Yet they carry important consequences: reduced work productivity, impaired relationships, increased healthcare utilization, risk of substance misuse, and the potential to evolve into chronic mood or anxiety disorders if not identified and managed proactively.

In contemporary societies, the prevalence of borderline, subthreshold mood and anxiety states appears to be rising or at least more visible. Epidemiologically, estimates vary by population and measurement method, but cross-sectional surveys routinely find that a substantial minority of adults report clinically relevant symptoms of stress, anxiety, or low mood that impair functioning without meeting full diagnostic criteria. This "clinical gray zone" is clinically important because it is both prevalent and amenable to early intervention—an opportunity to prevent progression to more disabling disorders.

Borderline disorders present diagnostic and therapeutic challenges. Symptoms are often nonspecific, fluctuate with life events, and overlap with somatic and sleep complaints. Standard psychopharmacology and psychotherapy remain central, but they have limitations in subthreshold conditions: pharmacologic agents may be unnecessary or poorly tolerated, while access to evidence-based psychotherapy is uneven and adherence variable. These realities create an opening for integrative approaches that combine psychosocial care with biologically targeted, low-risk interventions designed to restore homeostasis, enhance resilience, and correct underlying pathophysiology. Modern neuroscience and systems biology emphasize that mood and anxiety symptoms emerge from interacting networks, including the neuroendocrine (HPA axis), immune/inflammatory, neurotrophic signaling, neurotransmitter systems, mitochondrial and metabolic functions, and the gut–brain axis. Interventions that address only neurotransmitter imbalance may leave other drivers - such as inflammation, impaired bioenergetics, and dysregulated neuromodulators - uncorrected. A comprehensive strategy, therefore, combines psychosocial therapies and lifestyle medicine with targeted biological adjuncts that are mechanistically rational, personalized, and safety-minded.

Peptide-based therapeutics represent an emerging class of biologically active compounds with promising applications in modulating stress reactivity, emotional regulation, and anxiety. Neuromodulatory peptides, along with other small regulatory peptides, have demonstrated significant roles in influencing neuroendocrine signaling pathways that govern affective states, stress adaptation, and social attachment behaviors. These peptides act through specific receptor-mediated mechanisms, modulating neuronal excitability and network connectivity in key limbic and hypothalamic regions implicated in emotional regulation. Current evidence supports their potential use as adjunctive treatments rather than primary monotherapies, enhancing the efficacy of psychotherapeutic interventions. By improving emotional regulation, stress tolerance, and interpersonal engagement, peptide therapeutics may facilitate more favorable outcomes in individuals with borderline mood and anxiety disorders. Ongoing research aims to optimize their delivery systems, dosing strategies, and safety profiles to enable integration into individualized treatment protocols.

Organoid technology and mito-organelle's research provide a powerful translational platform for investigating the cellular and molecular underpinnings of neuropsychiatric vulnerability. Neural organoids - three-dimensional cell culture models that recapitulate key aspects of human brain development and function—allow researchers to study neuronal bioenergetics, mitochondrial dynamics, and cell-type–specific metabolic vulnerabilities with high precision. These models enable the identification of bioenergetic deficiencies and mitochondrial dysfunctions that may contribute to mood dysregulation, anxiety susceptibility, and stress intolerance. Moreover, organoid platforms can be utilized for the preclinical testing of novel biologic agents, including peptides and cellular modulators, enabling targeted and personalized therapeutic strategies. This approach represents a crucial step toward a mechanism-based approach, bridging basic neuroscience with individualized clinical interventions.

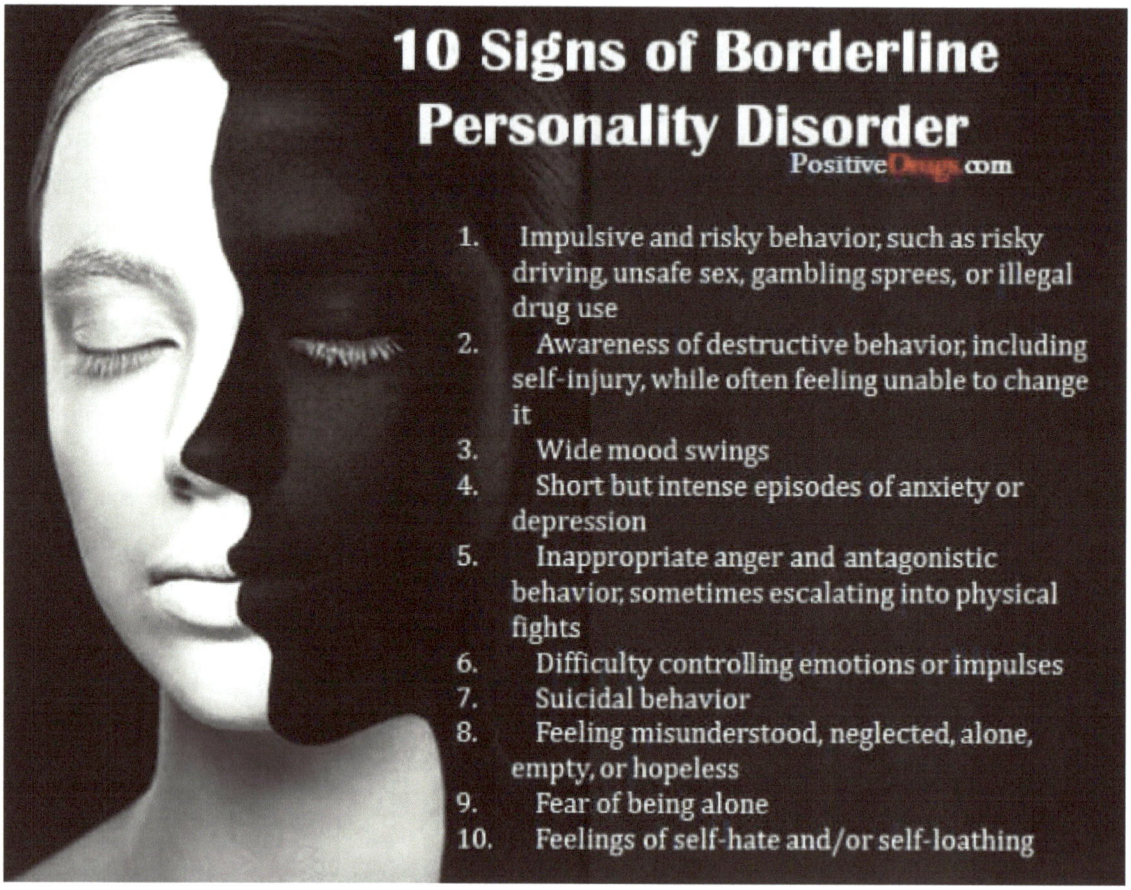

Source: positivedrugs.com

Cellular-based interventions offer another frontier in the biologically informed management of borderline mental disorders. Current strategies focus on modulating glial activity, including astrocytic and microglial functions, which play crucial roles in neuroinflammation, synaptic maintenance, and network homeostasis. Early-stage regenerative approaches aim to enhance neuronal support and resilience rather than pursuing unproven curative claims. Interventions that restore physiological balance in glial–neuronal interactions may reduce maladaptive stress responses and improve overall emotional stability. These methods may ultimately complement psychopharmacological and psychotherapeutic interventions, contributing to a more integrated model of care.

Physiotherapeutic and structured lifestyle interventions form a cornerstone of comprehensive care in borderline mental disorders. Evidence-based exercise prescriptions have demonstrated beneficial effects on neuroplasticity, stress regulation, and mood stabilization by modulating neurotrophic factors and neuroendocrine pathways. Specific physiotherapy protocols, including vestibular and proprioceptive therapies, target autonomic regulation and sensory integration, thereby reducing somatic manifestations of stress and anxiety.

Additional modalities include structured sleep interventions, breathing techniques, and movement-based therapies such as yoga and tai chi, which enhance vagal tone and promote emotional regulation. Noninvasive neuromodulation techniques can further augment these effects, providing synergistic benefits when combined with biological and psychotherapeutic strategies. Practical clinical algorithms guide the safe and individualized integration of these interventions, ensuring high patient acceptability and minimal adverse effects.

This book is written to bridge the gap between established psychiatric practice and emergent biological strategies for managing borderline disorders. Its aim is pragmatic and translational: to synthesize current science, present experimental and early clinical data, and provide clinicians and researchers with a roadmap for responsible, evidence-informed adoption of novel biologic tools alongside psychotherapeutic and physiotherapeutic care.

Borderline Mental Disorders—Definition and Understanding

Borderline mental disorders, most notably exemplified by borderline personality disorder (BPD), represent a category of psychological conditions characterized by marked instability in emotions, self-image, behavior, and interpersonal relationships. Individuals experiencing these disorders often feel emotions with heightened intensity and may struggle to regulate them effectively. The internal sense of identity can be fluid or fragile, shifting according to external circumstances or relationships. This instability can lead to sudden changes in views, goals, and self-perception, creating a sense of confusion or chronic emptiness.

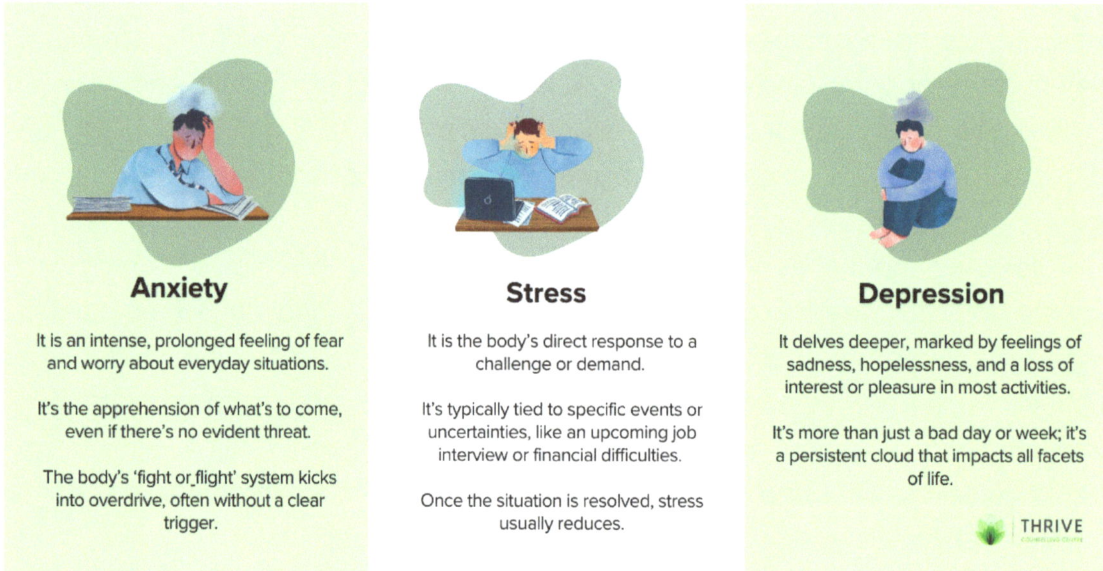

Source: Thrive

A central aspect of borderline mental disorders involves extreme sensitivity to perceived rejection or abandonment. Even small changes in social dynamics may trigger strong emotional responses, making relationships turbulent or unpredictable. People with borderline traits may deeply desire connection and closeness yet fear that others will leave them, contributing to patterns of clinginess, conflict, or withdrawal in interpersonal interactions. Emotional reactions that may feel overwhelming can sometimes lead to impulsive behaviors intended to relieve distress or regain control, although these behaviors can later be regretted.

From a cognitive standpoint, thought patterns in borderline mental disorders can shift rapidly, moving between idealization and devaluation of oneself or others. This polarized perception, sometimes referred to as black-and-white thinking, influences decision-making and social judgments. Additionally, a heightened reactivity to stress can momentarily disrupt a sense of reality or trigger dissociative experiences such as feeling disconnected from one's thoughts or surroundings.

Understanding borderline mental disorders requires recognizing the crucial role of emotional vulnerability and the difficulty in translating emotional experience into regulated action. These conditions do not reflect a lack of desire to function well or maintain relationships; rather, they stem from profound challenges in processing and expressing internal states. People affected often exhibit resilience, creativity, and deep empathy, yet they face ongoing struggles in navigating internal turmoil and interpersonal complexities. Borderline mental disorders, therefore, represent not a weakness but a different pattern of emotional functioning that requires understanding, patience, and structured support to foster stability and well-being.

Borderline mental disorders can be conceptualized through the lens of emotional regulation systems in the brain. Research highlights atypical activation in regions such as the amygdala, which rapidly detects emotional significance, and the prefrontal cortex, which modulates emotional responses. When regulation mechanisms are strained, emotions may escalate quickly and feel uncontrollable. This neurobiological perspective illustrates that the intense mood shifts seen in borderline presentations are linked to altered processing of emotional stimuli rather than intentional behavior or personality flaws. It emphasizes how deeply rooted these responses are in brain function and neural connectivity.

Interpersonal functioning in borderline mental disorders reflects a dynamic interaction between heightened emotional sensitivity and difficulty interpreting social cues accurately. Ambiguous facial expressions, tone of voice, or interpersonal changes may be perceived as threats, leading to rapid assumptions of rejection or hostility. This can result in misunderstandings that escalate interpersonal tensions, reinforcing the person's fear of abandonment. The pattern is not driven by a desire for conflict but by an urgent emotional need for reassurance and connection. These relational challenges often contribute to the chronic instability that characterizes the disorder across social and attachment contexts.

Self-concept plays a crucial role in the lived experience of borderline mental disorders. Identity may feel fragmented or constantly shifting, with individuals describing themselves differently depending on the situation, emotional state, or relational environment. This unstable self-image can affect long-term planning, career decisions, and a sense of personal continuity across time. Episodes of intense emotion can temporarily distort self-perception, leading to guilt, shame, or sudden changes in self-worth. The struggle to maintain a cohesive inner narrative contributes to a sense of internal confusion or disorientation.

Cognitive processing in borderline mental disorders often involves rapid transitions between contrasting beliefs or evaluations, particularly in interpersonal settings. A person may idealize someone during moments of positive connection and abruptly shift to feeling betrayed or devalued when discomfort or conflict arises. This cognitive pattern, sometimes referred to as splitting, reflects difficulty in integrating contradictory emotional information into a stable appraisal of oneself or others. These fluctuations can be exhausting for both the affected individual and those around them, yet they reflect an attempt to make sense of powerful and rapidly changing emotional experiences.

Stress

Stress is a natural physiological and psychological response to external demands or pressures. It activates systems in the brain and body that prepare a person to respond to threats or challenges, commonly known as the "fight, flight, or freeze" response. While stress can sometimes enhance focus, motivation, and performance, prolonged or excessive stress disrupts the body's balance and can wear down mental and physical functioning. Stress involves cognitive strain, emotional tension, and physical arousal, often accompanied by irritability, fatigue, and difficulty concentrating. Because stress is linked to how individuals perceive events, what overwhelms one person may be manageable for another. Over time, persistent stress can alter mood regulation and contribute to broader mental health difficulties, affecting sleep, appetite, and overall quality of life. It is an experience that lies at the intersection of environmental pressures and personal coping resources.

Stress operates on multiple levels, involving a complex interplay between the nervous, endocrine, and immune systems. When a stressor is perceived, the hypothalamic-pituitary-adrenal (HPA) axis activates, releasing cortisol and other stress hormones into the bloodstream. These hormones mobilize energy resources, heighten alertness, and prioritize survival-related functions. While adaptive in short bursts, prolonged activation can disrupt homeostasis, impacting cognitive performance, emotional regulation, and overall physiological balance. The neuroendocrine response illustrates that stress is not merely a psychological phenomenon but a holistic bodily process that integrates perception, emotion, and physiological readiness.

Cognitive appraisal plays a central role in how stress is experienced. The same environmental demand may be interpreted as a challenge by one individual and a threat by another, influencing both the intensity and duration of the stress response. Cognitive processes such as attention, memory, and expectation interact with emotional reactions, shaping the subjective experience of stress. For example, persistent rumination or worry can amplify physiological arousal and prolong the activation of stress pathways, demonstrating the interdependence of thought and bodily response. This emphasizes that stress is as much a product of perception as it is of external circumstances.

Stress also affects emotional processing and regulation. Heightened arousal can lead to irritability, impatience, or emotional hypersensitivity, reducing tolerance for minor frustrations and increasing conflict in interpersonal relationships. The amplification of emotions under stress reflects the brain's prioritization of rapid evaluation and response over reflective reasoning, particularly in regions such as the amygdala and prefrontal cortex. Consequently, individuals under chronic stress may perceive social cues as more threatening or interpret ambiguous situations pessimistically, further intensifying emotional distress. This feedback loop between cognition and emotion highlights why stress can feel both overwhelming and self-reinforcing.

The physiological consequences of sustained stress extend beyond immediate arousal, affecting cardiovascular, metabolic, and immune function. Chronic activation of stress pathways can lead to persistent elevation of heart rate, blood pressure, and inflammatory markers, which may indirectly affect overall health and cognitive functioning. Sleep patterns, appetite regulation, and energy balance are particularly sensitive to prolonged stress, as cortisol and other stress mediators disrupt circadian rhythms and homeostatic processes. Understanding stress within this broader physiological context highlights its role as an integrated mind-body experience, rather than a purely psychological state.

Finally, stress can have nuanced effects on behavior and adaptive functioning. In moderate amounts, stress can facilitate problem-solving, learning, and motivation, functioning as an energizing force that enhances alertness and performance. However, excessive or sustained stress may narrow attention, reduce cognitive flexibility, and impair decision-making. This dual nature illustrates that stress is not inherently negative but represents a spectrum of responses shaped by intensity, duration, and individual perception. Studying stress from this multifaceted perspective reveals how environmental demands, cognitive interpretation, and physiological responses converge to shape human experience in both adaptive and maladaptive ways.

Anxiety

Anxiety is an internal state of apprehension and heightened alertness that arises when the mind anticipates a possible threat or negative outcome. It differs from momentary fear by being more persistent, future-oriented, and often disconnected from immediate danger. Anxiety can affect the body through rapid heartbeat, muscle tension, restlessness, and an overactive startle response, while cognitively it can lead to excessive worrying, intrusive concerns, and difficulty controlling thoughts. Emotionally, anxiety generates uneasiness, dread, or a constant expectation that "something bad will happen." When anxiety responses are frequent or disproportionate to daily situations, they can interfere with decision-making, social interactions, and the ability to engage fully in everyday life. Anxiety shapes how one views the world, often magnifying uncertainty and making ordinary tasks feel like major obstacles. It emerges not only as fear of threats themselves but also fear of losing control over one's internal reactions.

Anxiety engages a complex network of neural circuits, primarily involving the amygdala, hippocampus, and prefrontal cortex. The amygdala acts as an early warning system, detecting potential threats and triggering rapid emotional and physiological responses. The hippocampus contributes to contextualizing these threats based on past experiences, while the prefrontal cortex is responsible for assessing risk and modulating the response. When these systems are overactive or poorly coordinated, individuals may experience persistent feelings of apprehension, even in the absence of immediate danger. This neurobiological perspective highlights that anxiety is rooted in normal brain mechanisms that become dysregulated, rather than being purely a matter of conscious worry or imagination.

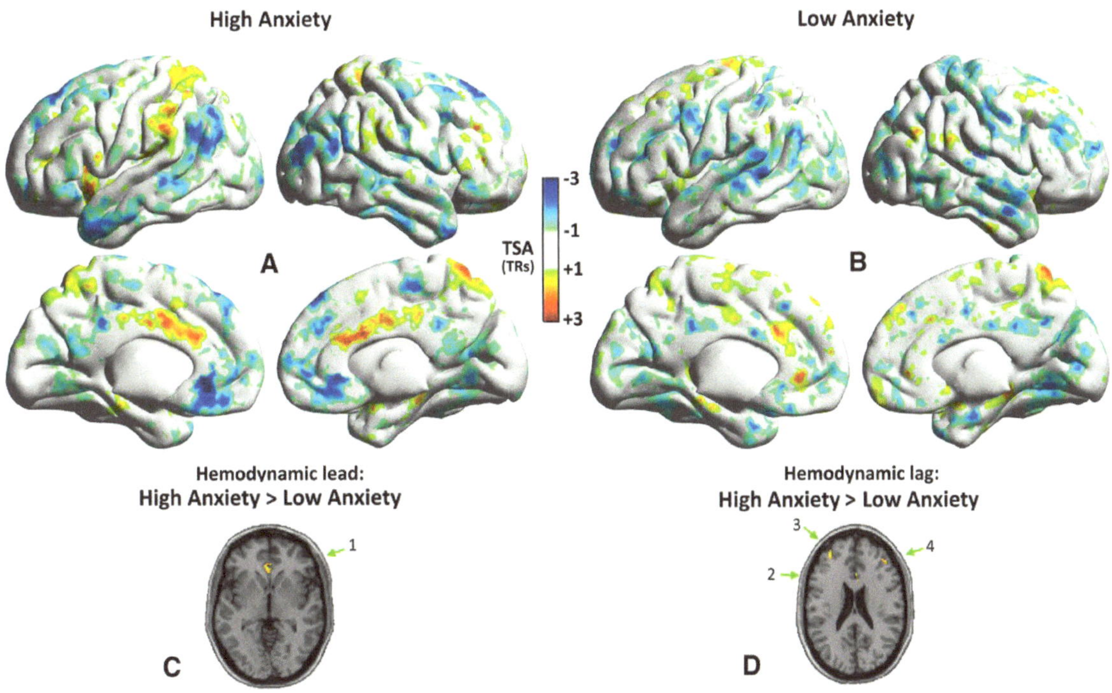

Whole-brain, time shift value maps in the subgroup of patients with NPSLE reporting significant anxiety symptoms (A; n=21) and patients reporting milder symptoms (B; n=11). Maps display voxels with haemodynamic lag (positive TSA values >1 TR) or lead (negative TSA values <−1 TR) within each group. Voxel clusters displaying significantly higher lead (C) or lag (D) in the subgroup of patients with high vs low depression symptoms are shown on appropriate axial views (independent-samples t-tests thresholded at p<0.001 uncorrected). The cluster displayed in (C) is located in the left subgenual ACC (1). Clusters shown in (D) are located in the right ACC (2), left (3) and right dlPFC (BA 46; 4).

Source: Antypa D, Simos NJ, Kavroulakis E, Bertsias G, Fanouriakis A, Sidiropoulos P, et al. Anxiety and depression severity in neuropsychiatric SLE are associated with perfusion and functional connectivity changes of the frontolimbic neural circuit: a resting-state functional MRI study. Lupus Science & Medicine. 2021

From a cognitive standpoint, anxiety often involves heightened vigilance and attentional bias toward perceived threats. Individuals may selectively attend to cues that signal danger, while filtering out neutral or reassuring information. This attentional pattern can intensify negative thinking loops, leading to persistent rumination and catastrophic expectations. Intrusive thoughts, difficulty concentrating, and memory interference are common manifestations, reflecting the brain's prioritization of threat detection over other cognitive processes. Over time, this heightened alertness can alter decision-making, making even routine choices feel burdened by uncertainty and risk assessment.

Emotionally, anxiety creates a state of sustained tension and uncertainty that differs from brief fear responses. Feelings of dread, irritability, and restlessness can dominate daily experience, often fluctuating in intensity without clear external triggers. The subjective perception of internal sensations, such as a racing heart or shortness of breath, can further amplify anxiety by reinforcing the sense of imminent threat. This cycle of heightened bodily arousal and cognitive vigilance demonstrates the integrated nature of anxiety, linking mind and body in a continuous feedback loop that can feel difficult to interrupt.

Physiological responses associated with anxiety extend beyond immediate arousal, influencing autonomic, endocrine, and immune function. Chronic anxiety can sustain sympathetic nervous system activation, increasing heart rate, blood pressure, and muscle tension. Elevated stress hormones, including cortisol, can disrupt sleep, energy balance, and immune regulation. These systemic changes illustrate that anxiety is not solely a psychological experience but a holistic physiological state that affects multiple bodily systems. Understanding anxiety in this context emphasizes its pervasive impact on both health and daily functioning.

Behaviorally, anxiety can manifest as avoidance, hypervigilance, or repetitive behaviors intended to reduce uncertainty. Individuals may limit exposure to situations perceived as threatening, seek constant reassurance, or engage in excessive planning. While these behaviors may provide short-term relief, they can inadvertently reinforce anxious patterns and narrow the range of experiences an individual is willing to tolerate. Importantly, these behaviors are expressions of underlying internal processes rather than signs of laziness or lack of resilience, highlighting the adaptive origins of anxiety responses that have become exaggerated or persistent.

Finally, anxiety serves an adaptive evolutionary purpose by enhancing survival in uncertain or dangerous environments. Moderate levels of anxiety heighten alertness, improve risk assessment, and motivate problem-solving. However, when anxiety becomes persistent, excessive, or disconnected from actual threats, it can interfere with daily life, emotional well-being, and social engagement. Studying anxiety through neurobiological, cognitive, emotional, and behavioral lenses reveals its multifaceted nature, showing how normal protective mechanisms can evolve into enduring patterns of apprehension that shape perception, thought, and action.

Depression

Depression is a mental and emotional state marked by persistent sadness, loss of interest, and a decline in motivation, often accompanied by changes in thinking, energy levels, and behavior. Unlike temporary feelings of disappointment or grief, depression endures over time and affects multiple aspects of daily functioning. Individuals experiencing depression may feel disconnected from activities or relationships that once brought enjoyment, and they may struggle to initiate even simple tasks. Thoughts can become dominated by feelings of worthlessness, hopelessness, or self-criticism, shaping a negative interpretation of oneself, the world, and the future. Physical changes can also occur, including altered sleep patterns, variations in appetite, and slowed movements or speech. Depression narrows a person's emotional experience, creating a sense of emptiness or emotional numbness where joy and fulfilment once existed. It is not a sign of weakness but a profound disturbance in mood regulation and internal drive that influences how a person thinks, behaves, and experiences life.

Depression involves complex interactions between brain circuits, neurotransmitters, and cognitive processes. Key regions include the prefrontal cortex, responsible for executive functioning and decision-making; the amygdala, which processes emotional stimuli; and the hippocampus, involved in memory and contextual evaluation. Neurotransmitter systems, including serotonin, norepinephrine, and dopamine, play critical roles in mood regulation, motivation, and reward processing. Dysregulation across these systems can contribute to persistent low mood, reduced motivation, and altered emotional experience, illustrating that depression is rooted in identifiable neurobiological mechanisms rather than a mere lack of willpower or resilience.

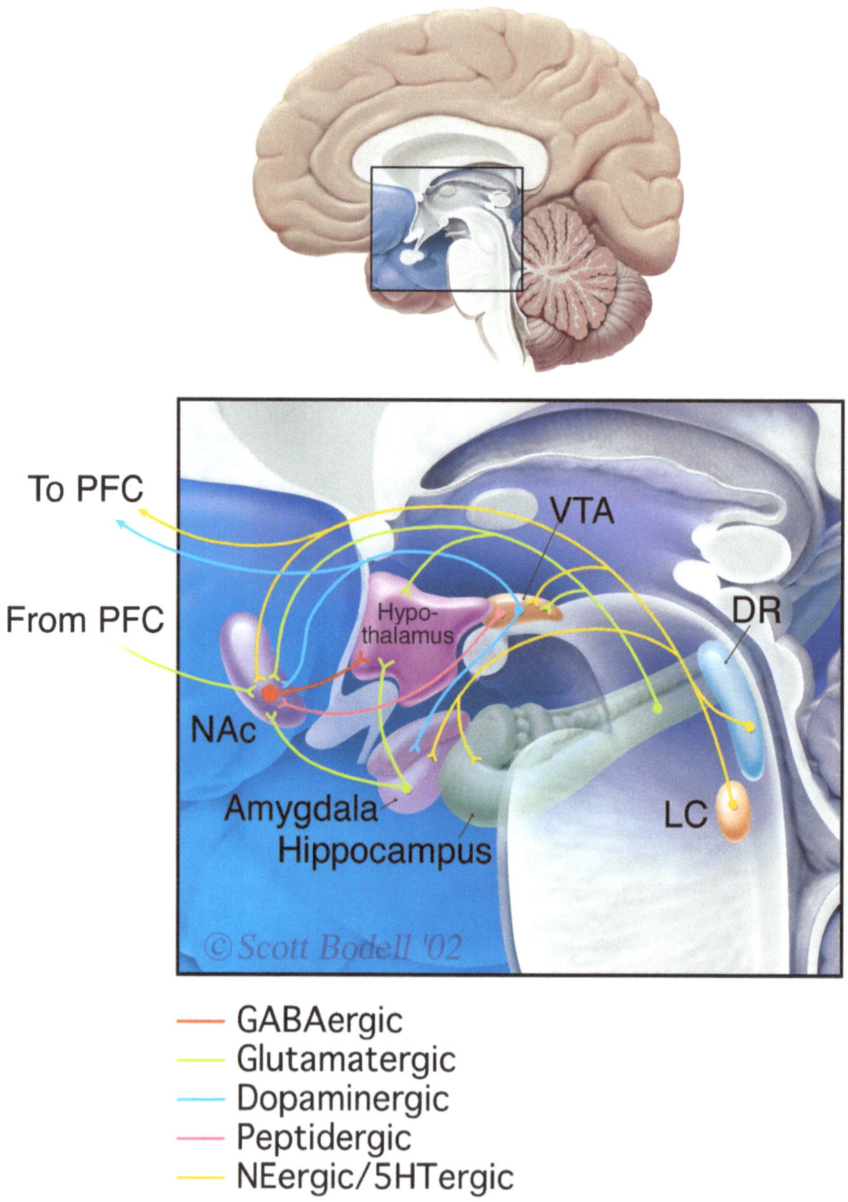

Neural Circuitry of Depression. Source: Eric J. Nestler, et al., Neurobiology of Depression, Neuron, Vol 34- 1, 2002

Cognitive patterns in depression often involve persistent negative biases in thinking. Individuals may interpret neutral or ambiguous situations pessimistically, ruminate on past failures, or anticipate negative outcomes in the future. These cognitive distortions reinforce feelings of hopelessness and self-criticism, limiting the ability to generate alternative perspectives or problem-solving strategies. Attention and memory processes can also be affected, making concentration difficult and reinforcing the sense of cognitive heaviness or mental fatigue that often accompanies depressive states. This interplay between cognition and emotion highlights how depressive experiences are both internally generated and contextually reinforced.

Emotionally, depression is characterized by a reduction in the ability to experience pleasure, known as anhedonia, alongside persistent sadness or emptiness. Emotional responses may feel muted, blunted, or dominated by feelings of worthlessness and guilt. The intensity of these emotional experiences can fluctuate, sometimes punctuated by brief moments of relief, yet the overarching tone remains negative and pervasive. This emotional narrowing affects interpersonal interactions, reducing responsiveness to social cues and diminishing the sense of connection with others. It demonstrates that depression is not only a mood disturbance but a disruption of the emotional landscape that guides daily experience and behavior.

Physiologically, depression exerts widespread effects on the body. Sleep disturbances, such as difficulty falling asleep, early waking, or hypersomnia, are common and can exacerbate cognitive and emotional symptoms. Appetite and energy regulation may also be altered, leading to weight changes, fatigue, or psychomotor slowing. Neuroendocrine changes, including alterations in cortisol levels, can affect stress response systems, while immune function may be modulated through inflammatory pathways. These systemic manifestations reinforce the idea that depression is an integrated mind-body phenomenon rather than a purely mental or emotional state.

Behaviorally, depression can lead to withdrawal, reduced activity, and diminished engagement in once-enjoyed pursuits. Daily routines may become disrupted, social interactions limited, and decision-making impaired. Individuals may struggle to initiate tasks or sustain effort, reflecting both the cognitive and emotional burdens of the disorder. These patterns are often interpreted as passivity or disengagement, yet they are manifestations of underlying disruptions in energy, motivation, and affective regulation. Understanding these behaviors within the broader context of depressive processes provides insight into the lived experience of the disorder.

Finally, depression can be conceptualized as a maladaptive extension of adaptive emotional processes. Low mood and withdrawal can signal the need for reflection, reassessment, or conservation of energy in the face of challenge. However, when these processes become prolonged or self-reinforcing, they evolve into patterns that impair functioning and quality of life. Examining depression from neurobiological, cognitive, emotional, physiological, and behavioral perspectives underscores its multifaceted nature, revealing how normal regulatory mechanisms can become dysregulated and give rise to enduring states of emotional, cognitive, and physical disturbance.

Integration and Conceptual Links

Stress, anxiety, and depression are intricately linked with borderline mental disorders. Heightened emotional sensitivity, cognitive biases, and physiological reactivity observed in borderline profiles intersect with stress responses, anxious vigilance, and depressive cognition. Neurobiological systems, including the HPA axis, amygdala-prefrontal circuits, and neurotransmitter pathways, provide a common substrate for these overlapping phenomena. Conceptually, these conditions illustrate how typical adaptive responses—emotion regulation, threat detection, energy conservation—can become dysregulated or intensified, giving rise to persistent mental health challenges. Studying these phenomena together illuminates the interwoven nature of emotion, cognition, and physiology in human psychological functioning.

The interplay between stress, anxiety, and depression in the context of borderline mental disorders can be understood through the concept of emotional reactivity. Individuals with heightened sensitivity often experience physiological and psychological arousal in response to minor environmental changes, which can amplify stress perception. This hyper-responsiveness may, in turn, trigger anxious anticipation of negative outcomes or exacerbate low mood, creating a cyclical reinforcement among stress, anxiety, and depressive symptoms. By examining these interactions, it becomes evident that the intensity of emotional responses is not isolated but shaped by cumulative influences across multiple psychological domains.

Cognitive processes serve as a critical bridge linking these conditions. In borderline mental disorders, polarized thinking, rumination, and attentional biases toward threat or loss can enhance vulnerability to stress, intensify anxiety, and perpetuate depressive cognition. These cognitive patterns influence how events are interpreted and encoded, shaping the subjective experience of internal and external stressors. For example, a perceived slight in a social interaction may simultaneously provoke emotional dysregulation, anxious anticipation of abandonment, and self-critical depressive thought, illustrating the convergence of cognitive, emotional, and behavioral dynamics in borderline profiles.

Neurobiological substrates further clarify the overlap between these conditions. The amygdala's role in threat detection, combined with altered prefrontal modulation in borderline mental disorders, contributes to heightened emotional reactivity, anticipatory anxiety, and difficulty regulating mood. Dysregulation of the HPA axis can prolong stress responses and influence neurotransmitter systems associated with depression, such as serotonin and norepinephrine. This shared neurocircuitry demonstrates that the co-occurrence of stress, anxiety, and depressive patterns is not coincidental but reflects converging neurobiological mechanisms that shape both emotional experience and behavioral responses.

Behavioral manifestations provide observable evidence of these integrated processes. Hypervigilance, avoidance, impulsive reactions, or social withdrawal may simultaneously express stress reactivity, anxious anticipation, and depressive disengagement. These behaviors, though often interpreted as maladaptive, can be viewed as extensions of normal adaptive responses to environmental demands that have become amplified or persistent. Observing behavioral patterns offers insight into the underlying emotional and cognitive dynamics, illustrating the interconnectedness of physiological, cognitive, and affective systems in shaping outward expression.

Finally, conceptualizing these conditions together underscores the importance of a holistic perspective in understanding human psychological functioning. Stress, anxiety, and depression do not operate in isolation; they interact with underlying personality structures, emotional regulation capacities, and cognitive processing styles to shape an individual's overall experience. Borderline mental disorders exemplify how heightened sensitivity and unstable self-concept can magnify typical adaptive responses, transforming them into persistent and impactful mental health challenges. This integrated approach emphasizes the interconnected nature of emotion, cognition, and physiology, providing a framework for understanding complex patterns of human psychological vulnerability and resilience.

Chapter 2

Epidemiology of Stress, Anxiety, and Depression: The Modern Mental Health Crisis

Global Prevalence and Demographic Patterns

A brief clarification regarding terminology: Borderline Personality Disorder (BPD) represents a distinct diagnostic entity from stress, anxiety, and depression, though substantial comorbidity exists. BPD is characterized by pervasive instability in interpersonal relationships, self-image, emotions, and marked impulsivity, rather than representing a "borderline" case of depression or anxiety as the name might suggest historically.

The prevalence of BPD is estimated at 1.6-5.9% of the general population, with higher rates in clinical settings (10-20% of psychiatric outpatients, 20% of inpatients). Contrary to the assertion in your question, there is limited robust epidemiological evidence for substantial increases in BPD prevalence over time, though improved diagnostic recognition may create apparent increases.

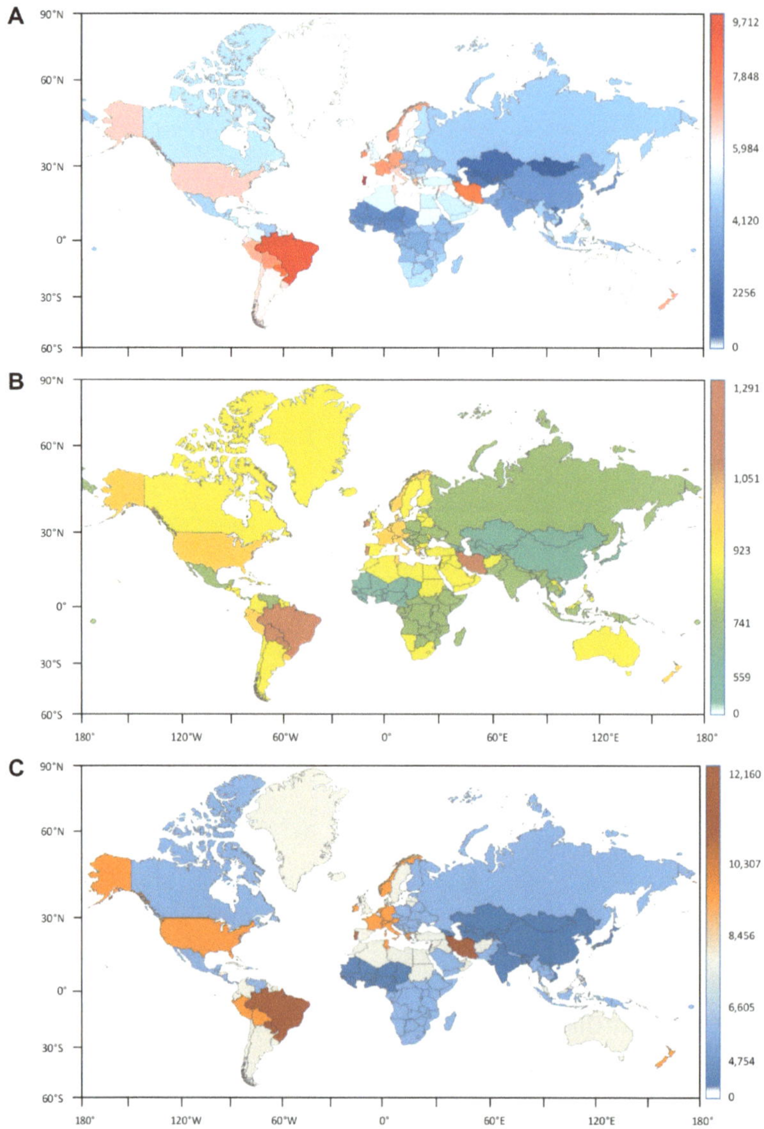

Age-standardized rates (per 100,000 population) of anxiety disorders in 204 countries in 2021. (A) age-standardized prevalence rates of anxiety disorders; (B) age-standardized incidence rates of anxiety disorders; (C) age-standardized DALYs rates for anxiety.

Source: Chen, Si et al. Dynamic changes and future trend predictions of the global burden of anxiety disorders: analysis of 204 countries and regions from 1990 to 2021 and the impact of the COVID-19 pandemic. eClinicalMedicine, Volume 79, 103014

What has increased is the recognition that BPD traits and emotional dysregulation exist on a continuum, and that subclinical presentations are common. The biosocial model of BPD development implicates interactions between emotional vulnerability (genetic/temperamental) and invalidating environments (childhood adversity, trauma). To the extent that modern environments are more invalidating or that developmental trauma has increased, one might hypothesize increased risk, though this remains speculative pending longitudinal epidemiological data.

BPD shows substantial comorbidity with depression (approximately 75% lifetime prevalence) and anxiety disorders (approximately 90% lifetime prevalence), and shares neurobiological substrates including amygdala hyperreactivity, prefrontal hypoactivity, and impaired emotion regulation. The chronic stress of living with emotional dysregulation contributes to comorbid mood and anxiety symptoms.

Depression

Major Depressive Disorder (MDD) represents one of the most significant contributors to global disease burden. According to the World Health Organization estimates, approximately 280 million people worldwide live with depression, representing roughly 3.8% of the global population. The lifetime prevalence ranges from 10-15% in high-income countries, with considerable variation across cultures and socioeconomic strata.

Depression demonstrates marked gender disparities, with women experiencing approximately twice the prevalence of men across most populations. This differential emerges during adolescence and persists throughout the reproductive years, suggesting contributions from both hormonal factors and psychosocial stressors related to gender roles. The peak onset occurs during early adulthood (ages 18-25), though depression can manifest across the entire lifespan, including increasingly recognized late-life depression in geriatric populations.

Socioeconomic gradients are pronounced, with individuals in lower income brackets, those with limited educational attainment, and unemployed populations showing substantially elevated rates. Urban-rural differences exist but vary by region, with some studies indicating higher rates in densely populated urban environments, while others document increased prevalence in isolated rural communities with limited access to mental healthcare.

Anxiety Disorders

Anxiety disorders collectively represent the most prevalent category of psychiatric conditions, affecting an estimated 301 million people globally (4% of the world population). This umbrella encompasses generalized anxiety disorder (GAD), panic disorder, social anxiety disorder, specific phobias, and separation anxiety disorder, each with distinct epidemiological profiles.

Generalized anxiety disorder affects approximately 3-5% of adults annually, with lifetime prevalence estimates ranging from 4-7%. Like depression, anxiety disorders demonstrate female predominance, with women experiencing rates 1.5-2 times higher than men. The age of onset varies by subtype: separation anxiety and specific phobias typically emerge in childhood, social anxiety disorder during adolescence, and GAD more commonly in early to middle adulthood.

Comorbidity patterns are striking, with 60-70% of individuals with anxiety disorders meeting criteria for at least one additional psychiatric diagnosis during their lifetime. The anxiety-depression dyad is particularly common, with approximately 50% of individuals with MDD also experiencing an anxiety disorder, and vice versa. This overlap has prompted ongoing nosological debates about whether these represent distinct entities or manifestations along a continuum of internalizing psychopathology.

Chronic Stress

Unlike depression and anxiety, chronic stress lacks a discrete diagnostic category in psychiatric nosology, yet its public health significance is substantial. Population surveys indicate that 55-75% of adults in industrialized nations report experiencing significant stress regularly, with 20-30% characterizing their stress levels as "extreme" or "barely manageable."

Chronic stress serves as both a risk factor and precipitant for numerous psychiatric and medical conditions, including depression, anxiety, cardiovascular disease, metabolic syndrome, and immune dysfunction. The allostatic load framework conceptualizes chronic stress as the cumulative physiological burden resulting from repeated activation of adaptive systems, leading to premature biological aging and disease vulnerability.

Vulnerable Populations and Health Disparities

Adolescents and Emerging Adults

As noted, young people demonstrate the steepest increases in depression and anxiety. Adolescent brain development, characterized by the ongoing maturation of the prefrontal cortex in contrast to earlier-developing limbic structures, creates a developmental window of heightened stress sensitivity and emotional reactivity. The overlay of modern stressors onto this neurobiologically vulnerable period amplifies risk.

Academic pressure has intensified, with college admission becoming increasingly competitive and student schedules incorporating multiple advanced courses, extracurricular activities, and standardized test preparation. The "achievement pressure" culture, particularly in upper-middle-class communities, correlates with elevated anxiety, depression, and substance use.

Puberty timing influences risk, with early-maturing girls demonstrating elevated depression and anxiety rates, potentially due to navigating sexual attention and relationship pressures before psychological maturity develops. Late-maturing boys face social challenges that increase their exposure to stress.

Racial and Ethnic Minorities

Racial and ethnic minorities experience disparate rates of stress-related conditions, though patterns are complex. African American and Hispanic/Latino populations report higher chronic stress levels related to discrimination, economic marginalization, and neighborhood disadvantage, yet demonstrate comparable or sometimes lower rates of diagnosed depression and anxiety compared to White populations.

This "epidemiological paradox" may reflect protective cultural factors (strong family networks, religious involvement, collective coping), differential help-seeking behavior, diagnostic bias (clinicians under-recognizing symptoms in minority populations), or genuine psychological resilience developed through adversity. However, minorities who do develop mood and anxiety disorders typically experience more severe, persistent, and treatment-resistant presentations.

The "weathering hypothesis" proposes that chronic exposure to social stressors accelerates biological aging in marginalized populations, manifesting as premature physical health decline. Racial discrimination represents a chronic psychosocial stressor associated with HPA axis dysregulation, cardiovascular reactivity, and inflammation.

Low Socioeconomic Status Populations

Poverty represents one of the most robust predictors of depression and anxiety. The chronic stress of financial strain, housing instability, food insecurity, neighborhood violence, and limited access to healthcare generates sustained physiological and psychological burden.

Children raised in poverty demonstrate elevated cortisol levels, altered brain development (reduced hippocampal and prefrontal volumes), and higher adult rates of mood and anxiety disorders. These effects persist even after economic circumstances improve, suggesting sensitive developmental periods where stress exposure exerts lasting impact.

The "deaths of despair" phenomenon describes increasing mortality from suicide, drug overdoses, and alcohol-related liver disease among working-class White Americans without college degrees, particularly in economically declining regions. This trend reflects the psychological toll of economic displacement, loss of community, and perceived status decline.

Neurobiological Vulnerabilities in Modern Contexts

Evolutionary Mismatch

Evolutionary psychiatry proposes that many contemporary mental health challenges reflect mismatches between ancestral environments that shaped human neurobiology and modern conditions. Human stress-response systems evolved to handle acute, physical threats where fight-or-flight responses were adaptive. However, modern stressors are predominantly chronic, psychosocial, and inescapable, for which these responses prove maladaptive.

Chronic activation of systems designed for short-term threat response produces the pathophysiological changes associated with depression and anxiety: HPA axis dysregulation, immune activation, metabolic dysfunction, and neurotoxicity. The modern environment thus represents a "mismatch" that chronically activates protective systems in contexts where their activation provides no adaptive benefit.

Similarly, social comparison mechanisms that evolved in small, stable groups now operate in contexts of social media exposure to thousands of individuals, many of whom are strangers, celebrities, or idealized representations. This scale exceeds the capacity of evolved psychological mechanisms to process meaningfully, generating maladaptive emotional responses.

Neuroplasticity and Environmental Enrichment

While human brains demonstrate substantial neuroplasticity—capacity for structural and functional change—modern environments may fail to provide the environmental enrichment that optimizes neurodevelopment and maintains mental health.

"Environmental enrichment" in neuroscience refers to conditions involving physical activity, cognitive stimulation, social interaction, and novelty. Laboratory animals raised in enriched environments show enhanced neurogenesis, synaptic density, and stress resilience compared to impoverished environments.

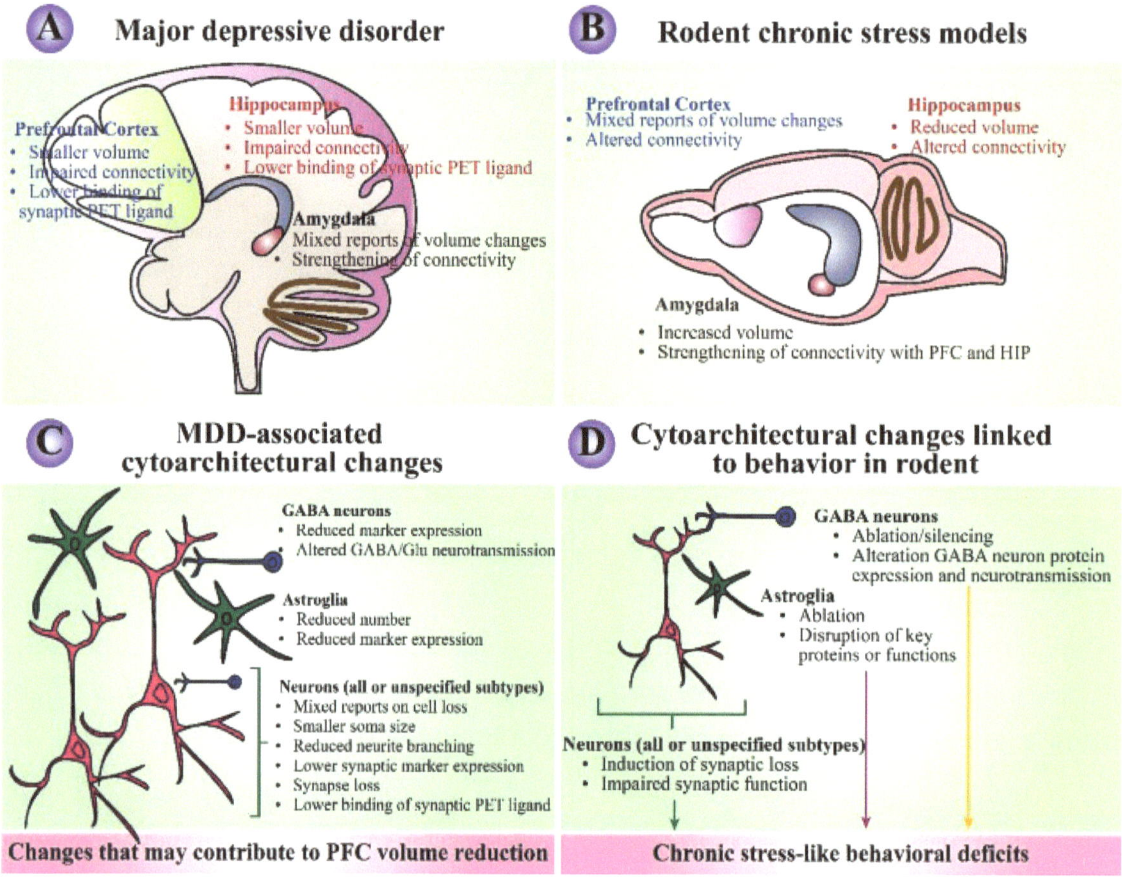

Source: Sami Awda Algaidi. Chronic stress-induced neuroplasticity in the prefrontal cortex: Structural, functional, and molecular mechanisms from development to aging. Brain Research, Vol 1851, 2025.

Contemporary lifestyles—characterized by physical inactivity, social isolation, repetitive cognitive tasks, and limited exposure to natural environments—may constitute relative "environmental impoverishment" compared to the conditions in which human brains evolved and develop optimally.

Public Health Implications and Future Directions

The Disease Burden

Depression represents the third leading cause of disability-adjusted life years (DALYs) globally, accounting for 4.4% of all DALYs across all diseases and injuries. Anxiety disorders contribute an additional 2.5%. Together, these conditions represent the largest psychiatric contributors to global disease burden.

Economic costs are staggering. In the United States, depression alone accounts for an estimated $210 billion annually in direct medical costs, workplace costs (absenteeism, presenteeism, disability), and suicide-related mortality. Anxiety disorders add approximately $42 billion annually. These figures underestimate total burden by excluding impacts on quality of life, relationships, and human potential.

The WHO estimates that for every dollar invested in scaling up treatment for depression and anxiety, there is a return of four dollars in improved health and productivity. Despite this favorable return on investment, mental healthcare remains dramatically underfunded relative to disease burden in most health systems.

Prevention and Intervention Considerations

The epidemiological patterns described suggest that effective prevention requires addressing social determinants of mental health: economic security, social cohesion, work-life balance, digital technology regulation, and built environments that facilitate community connection.

Individual-level interventions (psychotherapy, pharmacotherapy) remain essential but insufficient when environmental stressors continuously generate new cases. A public health approach requires "upstream" interventions addressing root causes rather than solely treating downstream consequences.

Promising population-level approaches include universal school-based prevention programs teaching emotional regulation and stress management, workplace interventions improving job control and organizational justice, urban planning prioritizing walkability and green space, and policies ensuring economic security (living wages, healthcare access, parental leave).

Conclusion

The epidemiological landscape of stress, anxiety, and depression in the 21st century reflects a complex interaction between biological vulnerabilities, psychological processes, and socioenvironmental contexts that differ substantially from conditions in which human psychology evolved. Rising prevalence, particularly among young people, suggests that contemporary life introduces novel stressors or removes protective factors that previously buffered against psychological distress.

The modern workplace, digital technology ecosystem, economic structures, social fragmentation, and information environment appear to represent significant contributors to this mental health crisis. While individual differences in vulnerability persist, population-level increases suggest that environmental changes are affecting broad swaths of society.

Addressing this public health challenge requires interventions at multiple levels: individual (enhancing coping skills and access to care), interpersonal (strengthening social connections), organizational (reforming workplace practices), community (building social infrastructure), and policy (addressing economic inequality, regulating technology, and funding mental health systems).

The neurobiological substrates of stress, anxiety, and depression—HPA axis function, limbic circuitry, and neurotransmitter systems—interact bidirectionally with environmental inputs, meaning that changing environments can shift population mental health trajectories. Understanding these interactions through rigorous epidemiological and mechanistic research will be essential for developing effective responses to one of the defining health challenges of our era.

Temporal Trends: The Rising Tide

Generational Increases

Epidemiological data from the past three decades reveal concerning temporal trends. Multiple large-scale cohort studies demonstrate substantial increases in the prevalence of depression and anxiety, particularly among younger generations. Birth cohort analyses indicate that individuals born after 1990 (Millennials and Generation Z) experience rates of depression and anxiety 30-50% higher than those born in the 1960s-1970s (Generation X and Baby Boomers) at comparable life stages.

Cross-sectional surveys of adolescents and young adults show dramatic increases beginning around 2010-2012, a pattern observed across multiple Western nations. In the United States, the National Survey on Drug Use and Health documented that major depressive episodes among adolescents (ages 12-17) increased from 8.7% in 2005 to 15.7% in 2020, representing an 80% relative increase over 15 years. Similar trends appear in collegiate populations, with the American College Health Association reporting that 41.6% of undergraduates experienced depression and 36.1% experienced anxiety in 2021, compared to 22.4% and 18.9% respectively, in 2008.

These generational differences persist even after accounting for increased awareness, reduced stigma, and enhanced diagnostic recognition, suggesting genuine increases in symptom burden rather than merely diagnostic inflation.

Global Variations

While the upward trajectory is most pronounced in high-income Western nations, emerging economies exhibit more complex patterns. Rapid urbanization and industrialization in countries such as China, India, and Brazil correlate with increasing prevalence of mood and anxiety disorders, though rates generally remain below those in fully industrialized nations. Cultural factors, family structure, social cohesion, and differential exposure to modernization stressors create heterogeneous epidemiological landscapes.

Low-income countries with traditional subsistence lifestyles tend to demonstrate lower prevalence rates, though methodological challenges in cross-cultural psychiatric assessment complicate direct comparisons. The "epidemiological paradox" describes observations that some populations experiencing objective material hardship report lower rates of certain psychiatric disorders than wealthier populations, suggesting that subjective experience, social support, meaning-making frameworks, and community cohesion may buffer against psychopathology in ways that material prosperity alone does not.

The Modern Life Hypothesis: Etiological Mechanisms

Digital Technology and Social Media

The proliferation of digital technology and social media platforms correlates temporally with observed increases in depression and anxiety, particularly among youth. While correlation does not establish causation, accumulating evidence suggests plausible mechanistic pathways.

Social media engagement promotes upward social comparison, where individuals evaluate their lives against curated, idealized representations of others' experiences. This comparison process activates reward circuitry while simultaneously generating feelings of inadequacy, envy, and low self-worth. Experimental studies have demonstrated that limiting social media use to 30 minutes daily results in measurable reductions in depression and loneliness scores compared to unrestricted use.

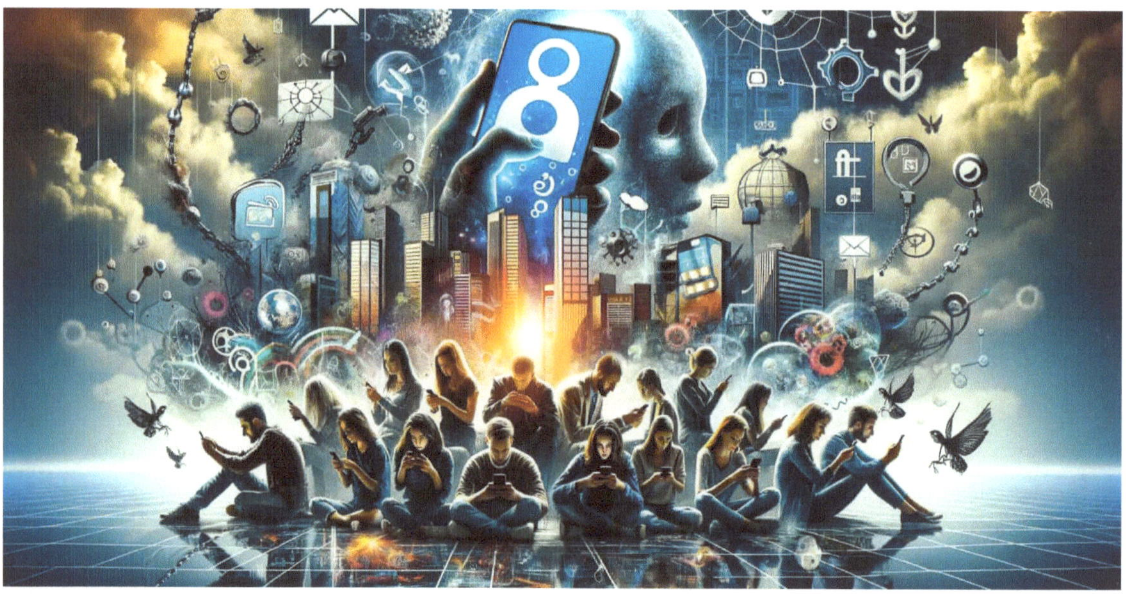

Source: https://www.psypost.org

The "fear of missing out" (FOMO) phenomenon describes anxiety related to perceived exclusion from rewarding social experiences others are enjoying. This psychosocial stressor maintains hypervigilance toward social information and perpetuates compulsive checking behaviors, disrupting attention, sleep, and face-to-face social engagement.

Cyberbullying represents a particularly pernicious stressor, as digital harassment is pervasive (accessible 24/7, invading home environments previously considered safe), permanent (content persists indefinitely), and public (visible to indefinitely large audiences). Victims demonstrate substantially elevated rates of depression, anxiety, and suicidal ideation compared to peers not experiencing cyberbullying.

Blue light exposure from screens disrupts circadian rhythm regulation by suppressing melatonin secretion, contributing to the epidemic of insufficient sleep among adolescents and young adults. Sleep deprivation represents a robust risk factor for both depression and anxiety, creating a vicious cycle wherein mood symptoms disrupt sleep, which further exacerbates psychological distress.

Atomization and Social Disconnection

Despite unprecedented connectivity through digital means, Western societies demonstrate declining rates of deep social connection. Sociological research documents a decline in community participation, religious affiliation, civic engagement, and spontaneous neighborly behaviors over recent decades. The number of Americans reporting having no close friends has tripled since 1990, from 3% to 12%.

Evolutionary perspectives suggest that humans evolved as obligately social primates requiring stable, supportive social networks for psychological well-being. The breakdown of traditional community structures—extended families living proximally, stable neighborhood ties, regular participation in collective activities—removes evolutionarily expected social scaffolding. This social atomization activates threat-detection systems, as social isolation historically signaled existential danger.

The decline of "third places"—community spaces distinct from home and work where informal social interaction occurs (such as churches, community centers, parks, and local businesses)—reduces opportunities for casual social contact that fosters community bonds and provides ambient social support. This architectural and urban planning shift toward automobile-dependent, privatized spaces contributes to isolation.

Economic Precarity and Work-Life Imbalance

Neoliberal economic restructuring over the past four decades has produced substantial shifts in employment patterns, compensation structures, and economic security. The erosion of stable, full-time employment with benefits, pension security, and predictable advancement pathways has created widespread economic anxiety even among employed individuals.

The gig economy and rise of precarious employment generate chronic uncertainty regarding income, scheduling, and future prospects. This unpredictability prevents long-term planning (purchasing homes, starting families) and maintains sustained activation of stress-response systems. Job insecurity correlates strongly with depression and anxiety, independent of actual income levels.

Work intensification—the expectation of producing more output in less time—characterizes many contemporary workplaces. Email and mobile devices blur boundaries between work and personal time, creating "always-on" cultures where disengagement becomes psychologically difficult. This boundary erosion prevents recovery from work stressors, promoting burnout characterized by exhaustion, cynicism, and reduced professional efficacy.

Income inequality has increased dramatically in most industrialized nations. Beyond absolute material deprivation, relative inequality itself generates psychological distress through status anxiety, perceived powerlessness, and chronic social evaluative threat. Societies with greater income inequality demonstrate a higher prevalence of mental illness, independent of average wealth levels.

The student debt burden in countries with privatized higher education creates substantial financial stress for young adults, delaying traditional developmental milestones (such as marriage, childbearing, and homeownership) and generating chronic worry about repayment. The average U.S. student loan debt has increased 300% since 2000 (adjusted for inflation), creating unprecedented financial strain on emerging adults.

Information Overload and Attentional Fragmentation

The contemporary information environment exposes individuals to exponentially more information than any previous generation. The average person encounters more information daily than a 15th-century individual would encounter in a lifetime. This information deluge overwhelms cognitive processing capacity, creating chronic mental fatigue.

Multitasking and rapid task-switching, encouraged by digital interfaces and workplace norms, fragment attention and reduce the depth of engagement. Research indicates that sustained attention spans have decreased, with implications for learning, relationship quality, and the ability to engage in reflective thought. The chronic sense of partial attention to multiple demands simultaneously generates background stress.

News cycles that emphasize sensational, threatening, and negative information (negativity bias in media) create distorted perceptions of environmental threats. Constant exposure to global crises, violence, and catastrophe—most of which individuals cannot personally influence—generates learned helplessness and existential anxiety. The 24-hour news cycle prevents psychological recovery between exposures to threatening information.

Decline of Meaning-Making Frameworks

Secularization and declining participation in traditional religious, spiritual, and philosophical communities have removed structured frameworks for meaning-making for many individuals. While individual freedom from prescriptive belief systems offers autonomy, it also places the burden of constructing existential meaning entirely on individuals.

The "meaning crisis" describes widespread difficulty answering fundamental questions about purpose, value, and significance in an increasingly materialistic, individualistic culture. Depression and anxiety often involve existential dimensions—meaninglessness, purposelessness, alienation—that contemporary secular societies provide limited resources to address.

Consumerism as a meaning substitute proves inadequate, as material acquisition provides only transient satisfaction and potentially undermines well-being through hedonic adaptation, social comparison, and the misallocation of time toward income generation rather than relationship cultivation and meaningful activity.

Environmental and Existential Threats

Climate change anxiety (eco-anxiety) represents an emerging phenomenon, particularly among young people who will live through accelerating environmental degradation. While not a clinical disorder, existential concern about environmental collapse, species extinction, and destabilized ecosystems generates chronic background stress, affecting reproductive decision-making and future-oriented thinking.

Political polarization and institutional distrust create perceptions of societal fragmentation and unpredictability. When institutions that traditionally provided stability and conflict resolution appear dysfunctional, individuals experience heightened uncertainty about collective futures.

The COVID-19 pandemic served as a massive collective stressor, with documented increases in depression and anxiety globally. Beyond direct health threats, social isolation from mitigation measures, economic disruption, grief and loss, and disruption of normal routines contributed to psychological distress. Many mental health indicators have not returned to pre-pandemic baselines, suggesting sustained impact.

The Modern Workplace: Occupational Stress Epidemiology

Burnout Syndrome

Occupational burnout has reached epidemic proportions across numerous professions. Characterized by emotional exhaustion, depersonalization, and reduced sense of personal accomplishment, burnout affects an estimated 50-70% of healthcare workers, 40-50% of educators, and substantial proportions of workers in corporate, service, and caregiving sectors.

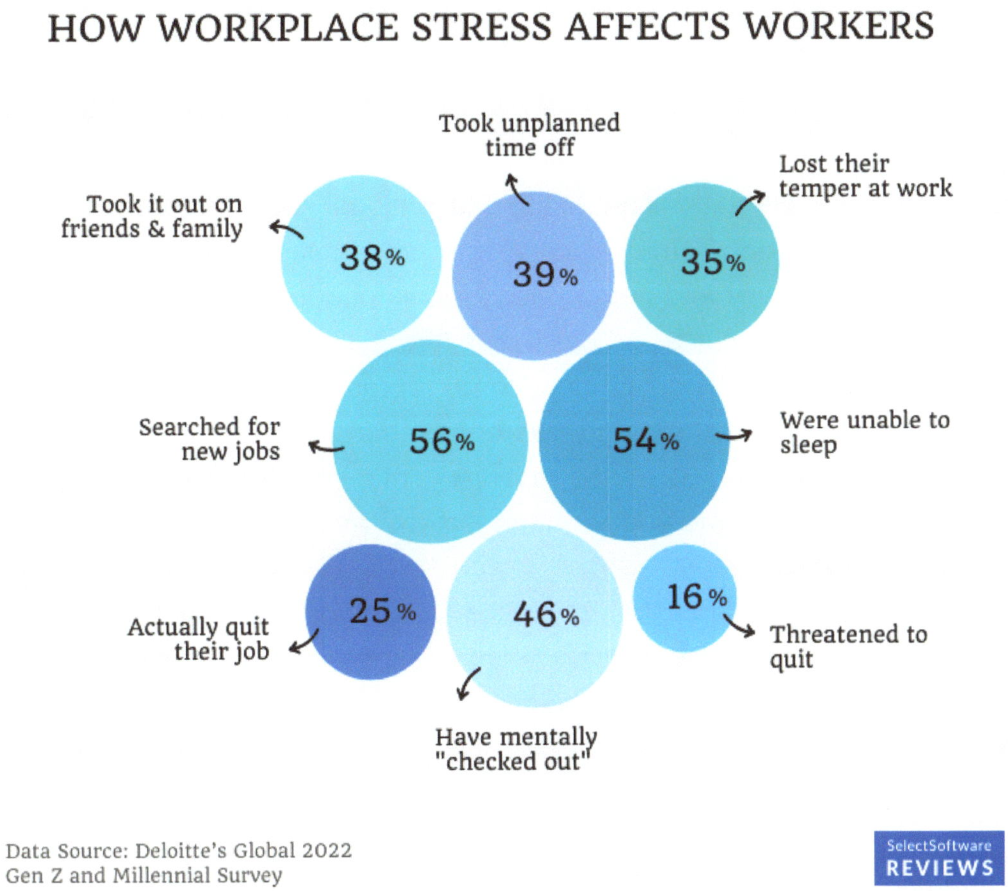

The Maslach Burnout Inventory, a standard assessment tool, reveals that emotional exhaustion—the core dimension of burnout—has increased significantly over the past two decades across various professions. Burnout strongly predicts subsequent development of clinical depression and anxiety disorders, representing a pathway from occupational stress to diagnosable psychiatric conditions.

Contributing factors include excessive workload, lack of control over work processes, insufficient reward (financial or recognition-based), breakdown of workplace community, perceived unfairness in organizational processes, and value conflicts between personal ethics and organizational demands. Healthcare systems operating under cost-containment pressures exemplify these dynamics, as clinicians face increasing patient loads, administrative burden, and ethical distress from rationing care.

Work-Related Anxiety Disorders

Specific anxiety presentations related to occupational stress include performance anxiety, meeting anxiety, email anxiety, and presentation phobia. The pressure for constant productivity and performance monitoring through digital surveillance technologies creates a sustained evaluative threat.

Job insecurity, as previously mentioned, represents a potent stressor. Even during periods of employment, the awareness that one's position could be eliminated generates chronic vigilance, inhibiting authentic workplace behavior as employees engage in "impression management" and avoid advocating for their needs or boundaries.

The "impostor phenomenon" or impostor syndrome—persistent feelings of fraudulence despite objective success—affects up to 70% of high-achieving professionals at some point. This psychological pattern creates chronic anxiety about being "exposed" as incompetent, despite evidence to the contrary, and correlates with perfectionism, overwork, and burnout.

Workplace Environmental Factors

Open-plan offices, despite their popularity for fostering collaboration, can increase stress through chronic noise exposure, a lack of privacy, constant interruptions, and a reduced sense of control over one's immediate environment. Studies indicate decreased productivity, increased sick days, and elevated stress hormones among workers in open-plan versus private office configurations.

A lack of natural light, sedentary work, and climate-controlled environments can disconnect workers from their circadian rhythms and physical activity, contributing to mood dysregulation. Office workers spend an average of 10-12 hours daily in indoor environments with artificial lighting, which disrupts their natural wake-sleep cycles.

Harassment, discrimination, and toxic workplace cultures generate substantial psychological harm. Microaggressions, exclusion, and hostile work environments particularly affect women, racial and ethnic minorities, and LGBTQ+ individuals, contributing to health disparities in stress-related conditions.

Chapter 3
Risk Factors

Risk factors for stress-related conditions, anxiety disorders, and depressive disorders operate across multiple levels of analysis, from molecular genetics to sociocultural contexts. These factors rarely operate in isolation; rather, they interact through complex pathways characterized by gene-environment interactions, developmental timing effects, and reciprocal causation. Understanding risk factors requires consideration of predisposing vulnerabilities, precipitating events, perpetuating mechanisms, and protective factors that modulate the expression of risk.

The diathesis-stress model provides a foundational framework: individuals possess varying degrees of constitutional vulnerability (diathesis) that interact with environmental stressors to determine whether psychopathology develops. This model explains why identical stressors produce varied outcomes across individuals and why some people develop disorders even with minimal apparent stress exposure.

Biological and Genetic Risk Factors

Genetic Vulnerability

Twin studies consistently demonstrate substantial heritability for both anxiety disorders (30-50%) and major depressive disorder (37-40%). This moderate heritability indicates that genetic factors contribute significantly but do not deterministically cause these conditions. First-degree relatives of individuals with depression demonstrate 2-3 times higher risk compared to the general population.

Molecular genetic research has identified numerous candidate genes associated with mood and anxiety disorders, though effect sizes for individual variants are typically small. Key systems implicated include:

- *Serotonergic system polymorphisms:* The serotonin transporter gene (5-HTTLPR) has been the subject of extensive investigation. The short allele variant is associated with reduced serotonin transporter expression, heightened amygdala reactivity to threat, and increased vulnerability to depression following stress exposure. However, this represents a gene-environment interaction—the short allele confers risk primarily in the context of adverse life events, not in their absence.
- *HPA axis genes:* Polymorphisms in genes regulating the hypothalamic-pituitary-adrenal axis, including the glucocorticoid receptor gene (NR3C1) and corticotropin-releasing hormone receptor genes (CRHR1, CRHR2), influence stress reactivity and recovery. Variants associated with enhanced or prolonged cortisol responses predict increased risk for stress-related psychopathology.
- *Brain-derived neurotrophic factor (BDNF):* The BDNF Val66Met polymorphism affects activity-dependent BDNF secretion, with Met carriers showing reduced hippocampal volume and increased vulnerability to depression and anxiety, particularly following childhood adversity.
- *Dopaminergic and noradrenergic genes:* Variants in catechol-O-methyltransferase (COMT), dopamine receptors, and norepinephrine transporter genes influence neurotransmitter availability and have been associated with anxiety sensitivity and stress reactivity.

Genome-wide association studies (GWAS) have identified hundreds of genetic loci associated with depression, each contributing minute effects. The polygenic nature of these conditions means that risk derives from the cumulative burden of many common variants rather than single high-penetrance mutations.

Epigenetic Modifications

Epigenetic mechanisms—including DNA methylation, histone modifications, and non-coding RNA regulation—mediate how environmental experiences influence gene expression without altering the underlying DNA sequence. These modifications can be transmitted across generations, potentially explaining intergenerational transmission of trauma-related vulnerabilities.

Early life stress induces persistent epigenetic changes in stress-responsive genes. Human studies document altered methylation of the glucocorticoid receptor gene in individuals exposed to childhood maltreatment, corresponding to heightened HPA axis reactivity. These epigenetic signatures may represent molecular mechanisms linking early adversity to adult psychopathology risk.

Importantly, epigenetic modifications demonstrate plasticity and can be reversed through environmental interventions, behavioral changes, or pharmacological treatments, providing potential therapeutic targets.

Neurobiological Vulnerabilities

- *Structural brain differences*: Neuroimaging studies reveal that individuals at high familial risk for depression or anxiety demonstrate structural differences prior to disorder onset, suggesting vulnerability markers. These include reduced hippocampal volumes, enlarged amygdala volumes, and altered morphology of the prefrontal cortex.
- *Functional connectivity patterns*: Resting-state functional connectivity studies reveal that individuals at risk exhibit altered connectivity within the default mode network, salience network, and frontoparietal control network. Specifically, heightened connectivity between the amygdala and ventromedial prefrontal cortex predicts stress vulnerability.

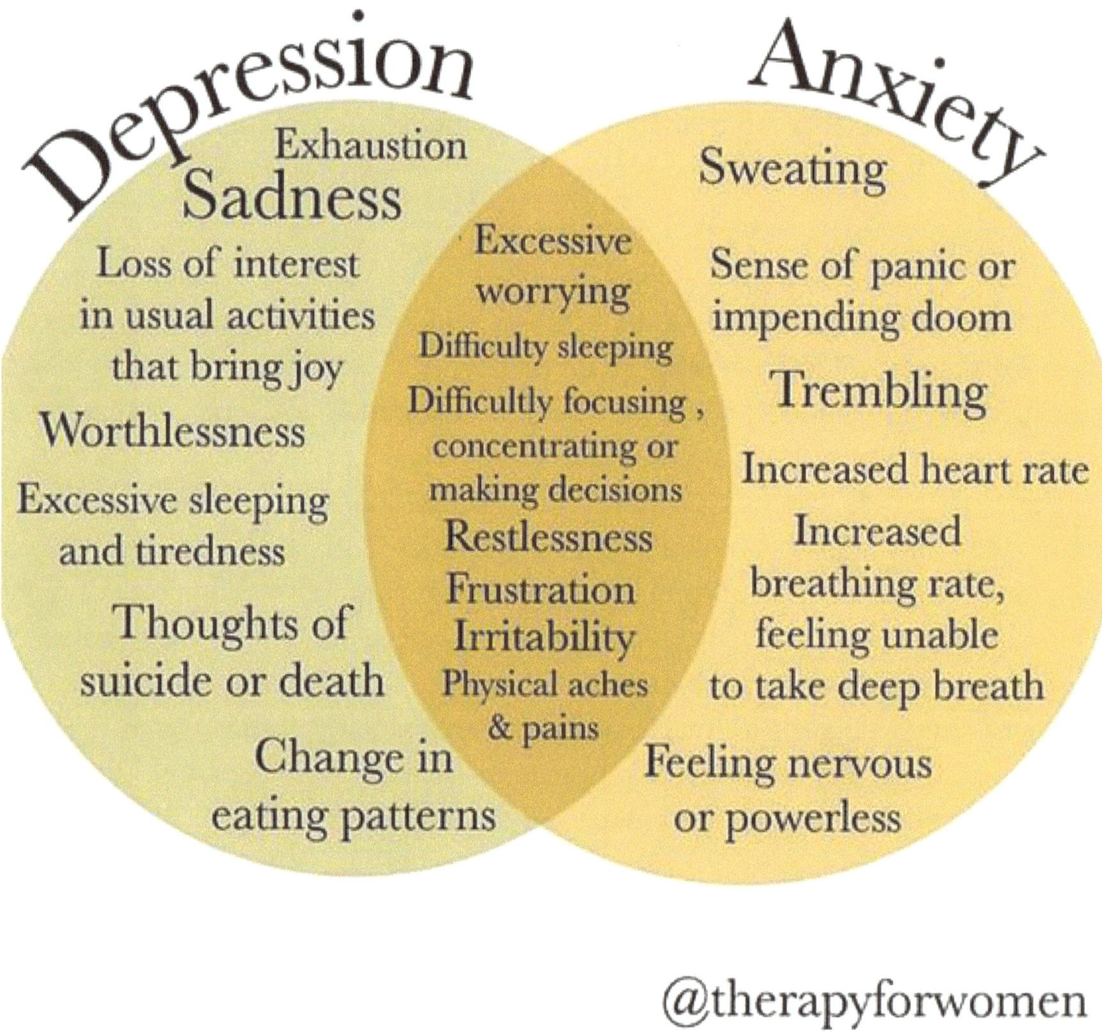

- *HPA axis dysregulation:* Some individuals exhibit constitutional hyperreactivity or hyporeactivity of the HPA axis, as measured by the cortisol awakening response, dexamethasone suppression tests, or cortisol reactivity to standardized stressors. Both excessive cortisol responses and blunted responses (potentially reflecting prior chronic overactivation) represent risk factors.
- *Inflammatory profiles*: Elevated baseline inflammatory markers, including C-reactive protein (CRP), interleukin-6 (IL-6), and tumor necrosis

factor-alpha (TNF-α), predict subsequent depression development. The "inflammatory depression" subtype demonstrates particular treatment resistance and may represent a distinct endophenotype.

- *Neurotransmitter system variations:* Baseline differences in serotonergic, noradrenergic, and dopaminergic function—measurable through neuroendocrine challenge tests, PET imaging of receptor densities, or CSF metabolite assays—contribute to vulnerability. Reduced serotonin synthesis capacity and altered receptor sensitivities increase risk.

Sex and Hormonal Factors

Female sex represents one of the most robust risk factors for both anxiety and depression, with approximately 2:1 female-to-male ratios for most disorders. This differential emerges during puberty and persists through reproductive years, implicating gonadal hormones.

- *Reproductive cycle influences*: Premenstrual periods, pregnancy, postpartum period, and menopausal transition represent times of heightened vulnerability. Premenstrual dysphoric disorder affects 3-8% of menstruating individuals. Postpartum depression affects 10-20% of new mothers, with onset typically within three months of delivery. Perimenopause is associated with a 2-4 times increased depression risk of depression.
- *Hormonal mechanisms*: Estrogen modulates serotonin synthesis, receptor expression, and monoamine oxidase activity. Progesterone metabolites interact with GABA receptors, influencing anxiety. Rapid hormonal fluctuations (as during postpartum or perimenopause) may destabilize neurobiological systems previously maintained at equilibrium.
- *Gender role stress*: Beyond biological sex, gender-related psychosocial factors contribute to the differential, including greater exposure to interpersonal violence, sexual trauma, caretaking burden, and gender discrimination.

Age and Developmental Stage

- *Adolescence*: This developmental period represents peak incidence for anxiety disorder onset and shows sharply increasing depression rates. Neurobiological factors include incomplete prefrontal cortex development, heightened reward sensitivity, enhanced peer influence, and hormonal changes. Psychosocial factors include challenges to identity formation, increased academic pressure, and navigating complex social hierarchies.
- *Early adulthood (18-25):* This "emerging adulthood" period shows high rates of new depression and anxiety onset, corresponding to major life transitions (leaving home, higher education, entering workforce, forming intimate relationships) occurring while neurobiological maturation continues.
- *Advanced age*: Late-life depression demonstrates distinct risk factors, including chronic medical illness, cognitive decline, functional impairment, social isolation, loss of spouse/peers, and reduced sense of purpose following retirement. Vascular depression, linked to cerebrovascular disease, represents a specific late-life subtype.

Medical Comorbidities

Numerous medical conditions substantially increase the risk for depression and anxiety through both biological mechanisms and psychosocial impacts of chronic illness:

- *Cardiovascular disease*: Myocardial infarction is followed by major depression in 15-20% of patients. Inflammatory processes, autonomic dysfunction, and the psychological impact of confronting mortality contribute. Bidirectionally, depression increases subsequent cardiovascular events.
- *Endocrine disorders*: Hypothyroidism, hyperthyroidism, Cushing's syndrome, and diabetes mellitus all demonstrate elevated psychiatric comorbidity. Thyroid hormones directly influence neurotransmitter

systems, while hypercortisolism mimics stress-induced changes. Diabetes involves complex management demands and complications that generate chronic stress.

- *Chronic pain conditions*: Fibromyalgia, chronic back pain, rheumatoid arthritis, and other persistent pain syndromes demonstrate 30-50% comorbid depression rates. Shared neurobiological substrates (including descending pain modulation pathways involving serotonin and norepinephrine) and functional impairment contribute.
- *Neurological conditions*: in cases of increased depression and anxiety risk through direct neurological damage, disability-related stress, and existential concerns.
- *Autoimmune and inflammatory diseases*: Systemic lupus erythematosus, inflammatory bowel disease, and rheumatoid arthritis demonstrate elevated psychiatric comorbidity, potentially mediated by inflammatory cytokines affecting brain function (the "cytokine hypothesis" of depression).
- *Chronic fatigue syndrome/ME:* This condition shows particularly high comorbidity with depression (50-75%), though causality is debated. Overlapping symptoms and shared pathophysiology (immune dysfunction, HPA axis abnormalities) complicate differentiation.

Psychological and Cognitive Risk Factors

Temperament and Personality

- *Neuroticism* – the personality dimension, characterized by emotional instability, negative affectivity, and stress sensitivity, represents one of the strongest personality predictors of both anxiety and depression. High neuroticism scores predict a 2-3 times elevated risk, which persists across cultures and assessment methods.

  Behavioral inhibition, a temperamental trait evident in infancy and early childhood, involves heightened reactivity to novelty, withdrawal from unfamiliar situations, and elevated physiological arousal. Behaviorally inhibited children demonstrate 4-7 times higher risk for developing anxiety disorders in adolescence and adulthood.

Harm avoidance, related to behavioral inhibition, involves excessive worry, pessimism, shyness, and fatigue. It correlates with serotonergic function and predicts anxiety disorders.

- *Negative affectivity* - the tendency to experience negative emotions intensely and frequently represents a transdiagnostic risk factor for both anxiety and depression.
- *Perfectionism* - particularly maladaptive perfectionism (setting unrealistically high standards, harsh self-criticism, excessive concern about mistakes) predicts depression, anxiety, and eating disorders. This trait generates chronic stress through unattainable self-imposed demands.
- *Dependent personality features* - excessive reliance on others for self-esteem and decision-making creates vulnerability to depression following interpersonal loss or rejection.

Cognitive Styles and Biases

Negative cognitive triad: Beck's cognitive model identifies three key negative schemas in depression: negative views of self (worthlessness), world (hostility/unfairness), and future (hopelessness). These schemas bias information processing toward negative interpretations. Repetitive, passive focus on negative emotions, their causes, and consequences (particularly common in women) amplifies and prolongs depressive episodes and predicts depression onset. Rumination maintains attention on distressing internal states while interfering with active problem-solving. Chronic, uncontrollable worry about multiple life domains characterizes generalized anxiety disorder but also represents a risk factor for anxiety disorder development. Worry may function as cognitive avoidance of more distressing emotions or situations. Anxiety-vulnerable individuals demonstrate automatic orientation toward threatening stimuli and difficulty disengaging from threat, measurable through dot-probe tasks and eye-tracking. This bias maintains hypervigilance and amplifies perceived environmental threat. Tendency to interpret ambiguous situations negatively or as threatening predicts anxiety. For example, interpreting physical sensations as catastrophic (common in panic disorder) or social ambiguity as rejection (common in social anxiety). Preferential encoding and recall of negative information characterizes depression. Depressed individuals more easily recall negative life events and interpret ambiguous memories negatively (mood-congruent memory). The expectation that negative outcomes are likely and positive outcomes unlikely, coupled with the belief that one cannot change this trajectory, represents a proximal risk factor for depression and suicidal ideation. Perceived inability to accomplish tasks or influence outcomes (related to Bandura's self-efficacy theory) increases vulnerability to depression following stress.

Emotion Regulation Deficits

Difficulty identifying, understanding, and modulating emotions represents a transdiagnostic risk factor. Specific patterns include:

Habitual suppression of emotional expression paradoxically intensifies emotional experience and physiological arousal while preventing emotional processing.

- *Experiential avoidance:* The unwillingness to experience uncomfortable emotions, thoughts, or sensations drives behaviors aimed at avoiding internal experiences, often at a significant life cost. This is central to many anxiety disorders.
- *Difficulty with distress tolerance:* Limited capacity to withstand emotional discomfort without engaging in impulsive or avoidant behaviors increases vulnerability to both anxiety (through avoidance reinforcement) and depression (through behavioral withdrawal).
- *Alexithymia:* Difficulty identifying and describing emotions correlates with depression and anxiety, potentially because it interferes with appropriate emotional processing and communication of distress.

Developmental and Early Life Risk Factors

Maternal stress during pregnancy: Elevated maternal cortisol crosses the placenta, potentially programming fetal HPA axis development. Children of mothers experiencing high prenatal stress demonstrate altered cortisol regulation and elevated anxiety. Maternal depression or anxiety: Independently of genetic transmission, maternal psychiatric symptoms during pregnancy predict offspring emotional difficulties, potentially through epigenetic mechanisms or intrauterine environment effects. Obstetric complications: Birth complications, prematurity, and low birth weight show modest associations with later depression and anxiety risk, possibly through effects on neurodevelopment. Prenatal substance exposure: Maternal alcohol, tobacco, or drug use during pregnancy affects fetal neurodevelopment, with associations to later behavioral and emotional problems.

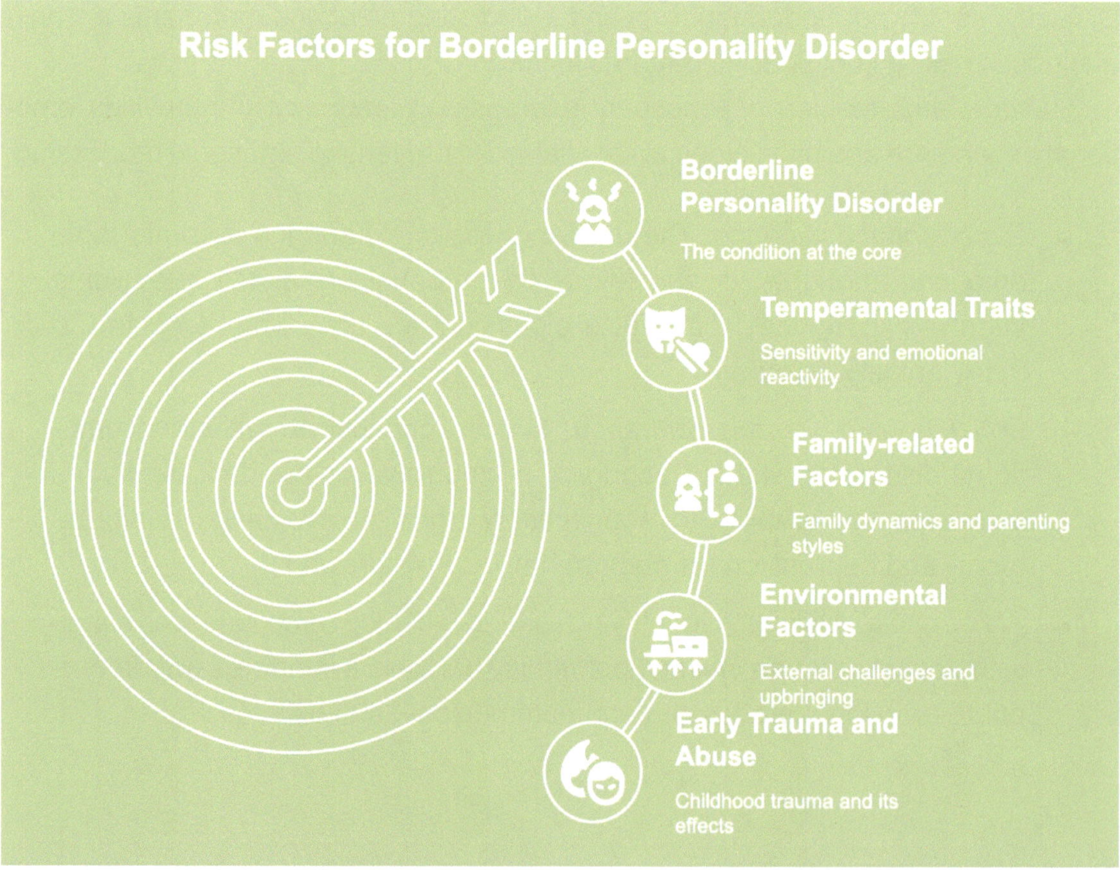

Source: https://diamondrehabthailand.com/

Childhood Adversity

Childhood adversity represents one of the most potent and well-documented risk factors for adult psychopathology. The dose-response relationship is striking: the Adverse Childhood Experiences (ACE) study demonstrated that individuals with four or more ACEs show 4-12 times higher risk for depression, anxiety, and suicide attempts compared to those with none. Experience of physical violence in childhood predicts adult depression, anxiety, and PTSD, with effects mediated through altered stress physiology, emotion dysregulation, and negative self-schemas. Childhood sexual abuse shows particularly strong associations with adult depression, anxiety disorders (especially PTSD and panic disorder), and suicidality. Effects appear partially mediated through shame, dissociation, and interpersonal difficulties. Verbal degradation, humiliation, and emotional cruelty produce psychological effects comparable to physical abuse. Emotional abuse particularly damages self-concept and emotional regulation capacities. Both physical neglect (inadequate food, shelter, and supervision) and emotional neglect (lack of affection, emotional availability, and responsiveness) impair attachment security and the development of self-regulation. Exposure to parental intimate partner violence functions as a traumatic stressor, even without direct victimization, through threat to attachment figures and chronic environmental unpredictability. The death of a parent, particularly before age 11 and particularly maternal death, significantly increases lifetime depression risk. Prolonged separation or parental abandonment produces similar effects.

Social and Environmental Risk Factors

Adverse Life Events

Acute stressful life events serve as triggers for disorder onset in vulnerable individuals. The relationship between stress and psychopathology is both causal (stress precipitating episodes) and consequential (psychopathology generating stressors through stress generation processes). Death of loved ones, romantic relationship dissolution, job loss, and miscarriage represent potent depressogenic stressors. The meaning attributed to loss and its impact on self-concept influences depression risk. Events involving loss of status, public embarrassment, or subordination show particularly strong associations with depression onset. These activate evolutionarily ancient defeat responses involving withdrawal and submission. Events involving an ongoing threat, physical danger, or situations perceived as inescapable predict anxiety disorders. The unpredictability and uncontrollability of the threat amplify anxiety risk. Academic failures, career setbacks, or sports defeats particularly impact individuals whose self-worth is heavily tied to achievement domains.

Chronic Stress and Chronic Stressors

Chronic stressors—ongoing difficulties that last for months or years—often have a greater cumulative impact than acute events. Poverty, debt, housing insecurity, and chronic financial strain represent powerful risk factors. The chronic nature of financial stress provides sustained HPA axis activation without resolution periods. Chronic marital discord, conflicted family relationships, or persistent interpersonal conflicts generate ongoing stress that predicts depression onset and maintenance. Job strain (high demands combined with low control), workplace harassment, job insecurity, and poor organizational justice correlate with depression and anxiety disorders. Providing care for chronically ill or disabled family members, particularly when resources are inadequate and the burden is heavy, substantially increases depression risk. Chronic experiences of racism, sexism, homophobia, or other discrimination function as persistent stressors with cumulative health impacts.

Social Support Deficits

Limited social network size, infrequent social contact, and perceived loneliness all predict depression and anxiety. The effect size rivals that of established medical risk factors. Absence of relationships characterized by emotional intimacy and the ability to discuss personal concerns increases vulnerability to depression following stress. Critical, demanding, or intrusive relationships can be more detrimental than social isolation. Quality matters more than quantity of relationships. Life transitions that disrupt established social networks (relocation, graduation, retirement) increase risk if new connections are not formed.

Trauma Exposure

Experiencing or witnessing life-threatening events, serious injury, or sexual violence can precipitate acute stress disorder, PTSD, and subsequently depression and anxiety disorders. Prolonged, repeated trauma (combat exposure, ongoing abuse, captivity) produces complex trauma presentations with extensive emotion dysregulation, identity disturbance, and interpersonal difficulties. Repeated exposure to others' trauma (common among healthcare workers, first responders, therapists) can produce secondary traumatic stress and burnout.

Lifestyle and Behavioral Risk Factors

- *Sleep difficulties* represent both a symptom and a risk factor for depression and anxiety. Insomnia increases depression risk two to four-fold, with the relationship likely bidirectional. Sleep deprivation acutely impairs the function of the prefrontal cortex, emotion regulation, and stress reactivity.
- *Circadian rhythm disruption*: Shift work, frequent time zone travel, and irregular sleep schedules disrupt circadian rhythms, affecting mood regulation. Social jet lag (discrepancy between social and biological sleep timing) correlates with depression.
- *Sleep apnea*: Obstructive sleep apnea, affecting 2-4% of the population, significantly increases depression and anxiety risk through sleep fragmentation, hypoxia, and inflammatory processes.

Physical Inactivity

Sedentary lifestyle represents a modifiable risk factor. Meta-analyses indicate that regular physical activity reduces depression risk by approximately 20-30%. Mechanisms include neuroplasticity enhancement (increased BDNF), modulation of neurotransmitters, anti-inflammatory effects, and improved self-efficacy.

Substance Use

Chronic heavy drinking directly increases depression and anxiety risk through neurotoxic effects, while acute intoxication and withdrawal produce mood fluctuations. The self-medication hypothesis suggests that substance use often begins as maladaptive coping, creating vicious cycles. Regular cannabis use, particularly high-potency products and use beginning in adolescence, shows associations with increased anxiety and depression risk in prospective studies, though causality remains debated. Cocaine, methamphetamine, and excessive caffeine can precipitate or exacerbate anxiety, while withdrawal produces depression. Chronic benzodiazepine use is associated with depression, possibly through neuroadaptation or as a marker of underlying anxiety severity.

Diet and Nutrition

Mediterranean diet patterns (high in fruits, vegetables, whole grains, fish, olive oil) show inverse associations with depression. Western diet patterns (high in processed foods, refined sugars, saturated fats) correlate with increased risk. Deficiencies in omega-3 fatty acids, B vitamins (particularly B12 and folate), vitamin D, magnesium, zinc, and iron have been linked to depression and anxiety, though causality is complex. Emerging research suggests that gut microbiota composition influences brain function through the gut-brain axis, with dysbiosis potentially contributing to mood and anxiety disorders.

Digital Technology Use

High daily screen time, particularly passive consumption and late evening use, correlates with depression and anxiety in both adolescents and adults. Frequency and duration of social media engagement show dose-response relationships with depression and anxiety. Mechanisms include social comparison, FOMO, cyberbullying, and sleep displacement. Internet addiction or problematic use patterns predict subsequent mental health deterioration, though directionality is complex (does internet use cause symptoms or do symptomatic individuals seek internet escape?).

Chapter 4

Classification of Stress, Anxiety, and Depression

The classification of stress-related conditions, anxiety disorders, and depressive disorders relies primarily on two major nosological systems: the Diagnostic and Statistical Manual of Mental Disorders, Fifth Edition, Text Revision (DSM-5-TR), published by the American Psychiatric Association, and the International Classification of Diseases, Eleventh Revision (ICD-11), published by the World Health Organization. These systems provide standardized diagnostic criteria that facilitate clinical communication, research comparability, and epidemiological surveillance.

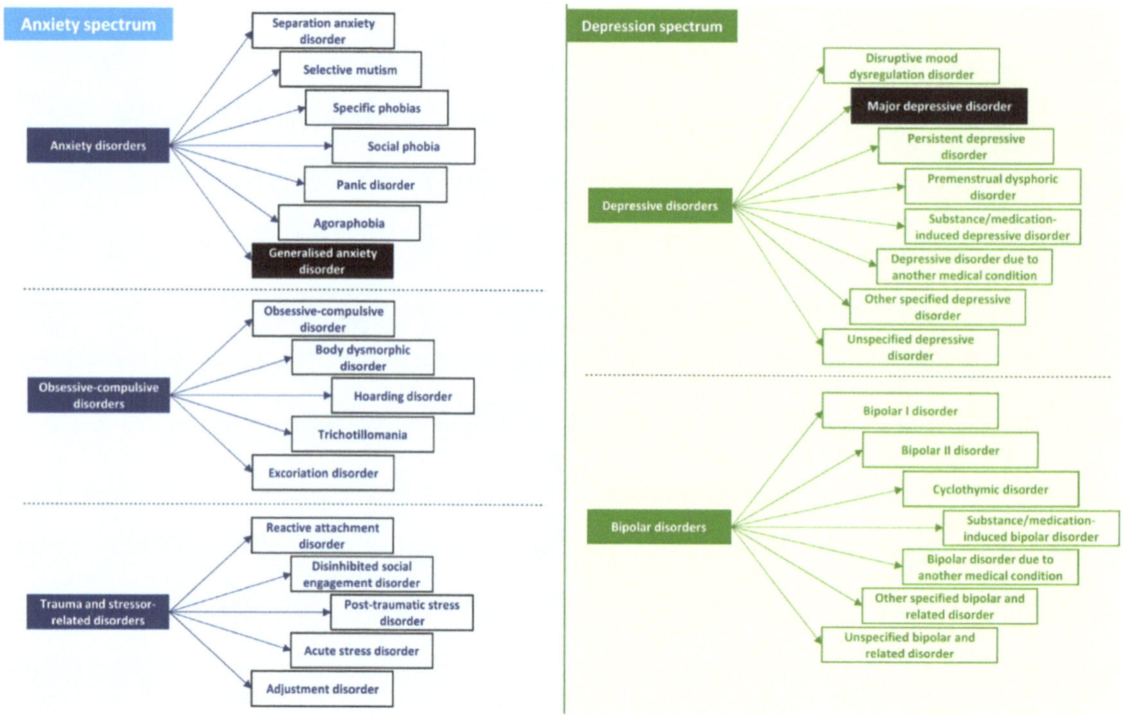

Source: Goodwin, Guy & Stein, Dan. (2021). Generalised Anxiety Disorder and Depression: Contemporary Treatment Approaches. Advances in Therapy.

Both classification systems employ a categorical approach, defining discrete diagnostic entities based on symptom clusters, duration criteria, and functional impairment thresholds. However, substantial overlap exists among these conditions, leading to ongoing debates about whether they represent truly distinct entities or dimensional variations along continuous spectra of psychopathology. Comorbidity rates exceeding 50% between anxiety and depressive disorders suggest shared underlying mechanisms and challenge strict categorical boundaries.

Stress-related disorders

Acute Stress Disorder (ASD)

Acute Stress Disorder represents an immediate psychological response to traumatic exposure, developing within three days to one month following the trauma.

The diagnostic framework requires exposure to actual or threatened death, serious injury, or sexual violation through direct experience, witnessing, learning that it occurred to a close associate, or repeated exposure to aversive details (as in first responders).

The symptom profile encompasses nine or more symptoms from five categories: intrusion symptoms (recurrent distressing memories, nightmares, dissociative reactions such as flashbacks), negative mood (inability to experience positive emotions), dissociative symptoms (altered sense of reality, inability to remember aspects of the trauma), avoidance symptoms (efforts to avoid distressing memories or external reminders), and arousal symptoms (sleep disturbance, irritability, hypervigilance, concentration problems, exaggerated startle response).

Symptoms must cause clinically significant distress or functional impairment and persist for three days to one month post-trauma. If symptoms extend beyond one month, the diagnosis typically transitions to Post-Traumatic Stress Disorder. The inclusion of ASD in psychiatric nosology reflects recognition that immediate post-trauma responses, while often resolving spontaneously, warrant clinical attention to prevent chronic sequelae.

Post-Traumatic Stress Disorder (PTSD)

Post-Traumatic Stress Disorder shares the traumatic exposure requirement with ASD but differs in temporal course, persisting beyond one month and potentially lasting years or decades. The DSM-5-TR organizes PTSD symptoms into four clusters rather than ASD's five.

Intrusion symptoms include recurrent involuntary distressing memories, traumatic nightmares, dissociative reactions (flashbacks ranging from brief episodes to complete loss of awareness of present surroundings), intense psychological distress at trauma reminders, and marked physiological reactions to trauma cues. At least one intrusion symptom is required.

Avoidance symptoms involve effortful avoidance of trauma-related thoughts or feelings and avoidance of external reminders (people, places, conversations, activities, objects, situations). Both avoidance criteria or at least one must be present.

Negative alterations in cognition and mood include inability to remember important aspects of the trauma (dissociative amnesia), persistent exaggerated negative beliefs about oneself or the world, persistent distorted cognitions about trauma causes leading to self-blame, persistent negative emotional state, markedly diminished interest in activities, feelings of detachment from others, and persistent inability to experience positive emotions. At least two symptoms from this cluster are required.

Alterations in arousal and reactivity encompass irritability or aggression, reckless or self-destructive behavior, hypervigilance, exaggerated startle response, concentration problems, and sleep disturbance. Two or more symptoms are required.

The diagnosis requires symptoms persisting for more than one month, causing significant distress or impairment, and not attributable to substances or medical conditions. Specifiers include "with dissociative symptoms" (depersonalization or derealization) and "with delayed expression" (full criteria not met until at least six months post-trauma).

PTSD exhibits substantial heterogeneity in presentation, with 636,120 possible symptom combinations meeting diagnostic criteria due to its polythetic structure. This heterogeneity has prompted research into PTSD subtypes, including proposals for a "complex PTSD" variant following prolonged trauma characterized by additional disturbances in self-organization (affect dysregulation, negative self-concept, interpersonal difficulties).

Anxiety Disorders

Anxiety disorders share features of excessive fear and anxiety and related behavioral disturbances. Fear represents the emotional response to real or perceived imminent threat, while anxiety involves the anticipation of future threat. These disorders differ based on the objects or situations that induce fear, anxiety, or avoidance, and the associated cognitive ideation.

Generalized Anxiety Disorder (GAD)

Generalized Anxiety Disorder involves excessive anxiety and worry about multiple events or activities, occurring more days than not for at least six months. The individual finds it difficult to control the worry, which is associated with three or more of the following symptoms (only one in children): restlessness or feeling keyed up or on edge, being easily fatigued, difficulty concentrating or mind going blank, irritability, muscle tension, and sleep disturbance.

The anxiety and worry cause clinically significant distress or impairment and are not attributable to substances, medical conditions, or better explained by another mental disorder. The content of worry in GAD is not confined to specific situations but shifts across multiple life domains (work, health, finances, family) in a manner that the individual experiences as uncontrollable.

GAD represents the anxiety disorder most closely associated with the personality dimension of neuroticism and demonstrates particularly high comorbidity with major depression, leading some researchers to question whether they represent distinct conditions or manifestations of a broader internalizing dimension of psychopathology.

Panic Disorder

Panic Disorder is characterized by recurrent unexpected panic attacks followed by at least one month of persistent concern about additional attacks, worry about attack implications or consequences, or significant maladaptive behavioral change related to the attacks (such as avoidance of exercise or unfamiliar situations).

A panic attack constitutes an abrupt surge of intense fear or discomfort reaching peak intensity within minutes, during which four or more of thirteen symptoms occur: palpitations or accelerated heart rate, sweating, trembling or shaking, sensations of shortness of breath or smothering, feelings of choking, chest pain or discomfort, nausea or abdominal distress, feeling dizzy or lightheaded, chills or heat sensations, paresthesias (numbness or tingling), derealization (feelings of unreality) or depersonalization (being detached from oneself), fear of losing control or "going crazy," and fear of dying.

Panic attacks are not limited to panic disorder and can occur in the context of other mental disorders. The diagnosis of panic disorder specifically requires unexpected (uncued) attacks not clearly tied to situational triggers, though situational attacks often develop subsequently. The phenomenology often involves catastrophic misinterpretation of bodily sensations—interpreting a racing heart as an impending heart attack, or breathlessness as suffocation.

Agoraphobia

Agoraphobia involves marked fear or anxiety about two or more of five situations: using public transportation, being in open spaces, being in enclosed spaces, standing in line or being in a crowd, and being outside the home alone. The individual fears these situations because of thoughts that escape might be difficult or help unavailable should panic-like symptoms or other incapacitating or embarrassing symptoms develop.

The agoraphobic situations almost always provoke fear or anxiety, are actively avoided or require the presence of a companion, or are endured with intense fear or anxiety. The fear or anxiety is out of proportion to actual danger and persists for at least six months, causing clinically significant distress or impairment.

While agoraphobia frequently accompanies panic disorder, it can occur independently. The cognitive model emphasizes fear of fear itself—anxiety about experiencing panic symptoms in situations where such experience would be particularly distressing or escape difficult. This metacognitive anxiety drives progressive behavioral restriction, potentially culminating in complete inability to leave home.

Social Anxiety Disorder (Social Phobia)

Social Anxiety Disorder involves marked fear or anxiety about social situations in which the individual is exposed to possible scrutiny by others. Examples include social interactions (such as conversations and meeting unfamiliar people), being observed (while eating and drinking), and performing before others (such as giving speeches). The individual fears acting in ways or showing anxiety symptoms that will be negatively evaluated, leading to rejection or offense to others.

Social situations almost always provoke fear or anxiety, are avoided or endured with intense distress, and the fear is out of proportion to actual threat. Symptoms persist for at least six months and cause significant impairment. A "performance only" specifier applies when fear is restricted to public speaking or performing.

Social anxiety disorder must be distinguished from normal shyness, which does not cause significant avoidance or distress. The disorder often manifests in adolescence, coinciding with the increased salience of peer relationships and social evaluation. Cognitive models emphasize exaggerated perception of performance standards, attention bias toward potential negative evaluation, and post-event rumination about perceived social failures.

Specific Phobia

Specific Phobia involves marked fear or anxiety about a specific object or situation that almost always provokes immediate fear or anxiety, is actively avoided or endured with intense distress, is out of proportion to actual danger, persists for at least six months, and causes clinically significant distress or impairment.

The DSM-5-TR provides specifiers for phobia type:

- **Animal** (spiders, insects, dogs)
- **Natural environment** (heights, storms, water)
- **Blood-injection-injury** (needles, invasive medical procedures)
- **Situational** (airplanes, elevators, enclosed spaces)
- **Other** (situations leading to choking, vomiting, in children, loud sounds or costumed characters)

The blood-injection-injury subtype exhibits a unique physiology—a diphasic response involving initial sympathetic activation followed by a vasovagal response (parasympathetic surge), which can produce bradycardia and potentially result in fainting. This distinguishes it from other phobias characterized by sustained sympathetic activation.

Specific phobias are among the most prevalent anxiety disorders, but often do not present for treatment unless the phobic stimulus is unavoidable or significantly life-limiting. Many individuals manage through simple avoidance without functional impairment reaching clinical thresholds.

Separation Anxiety Disorder

While most common in childhood, Separation Anxiety Disorder can occur across the lifespan. The disorder involves developmentally inappropriate and excessive fear or anxiety concerning separation from attachment figures, manifested by at least three of eight symptoms: distress when anticipating or experiencing separation, worry about losing attachment figures or harm befalling them, worry about events causing separation, reluctance to go places due to separation fears, fear of being alone, reluctance to sleep away from attachment figures, nightmares involving separation themes, and physical symptoms when separation occurs or is anticipated.

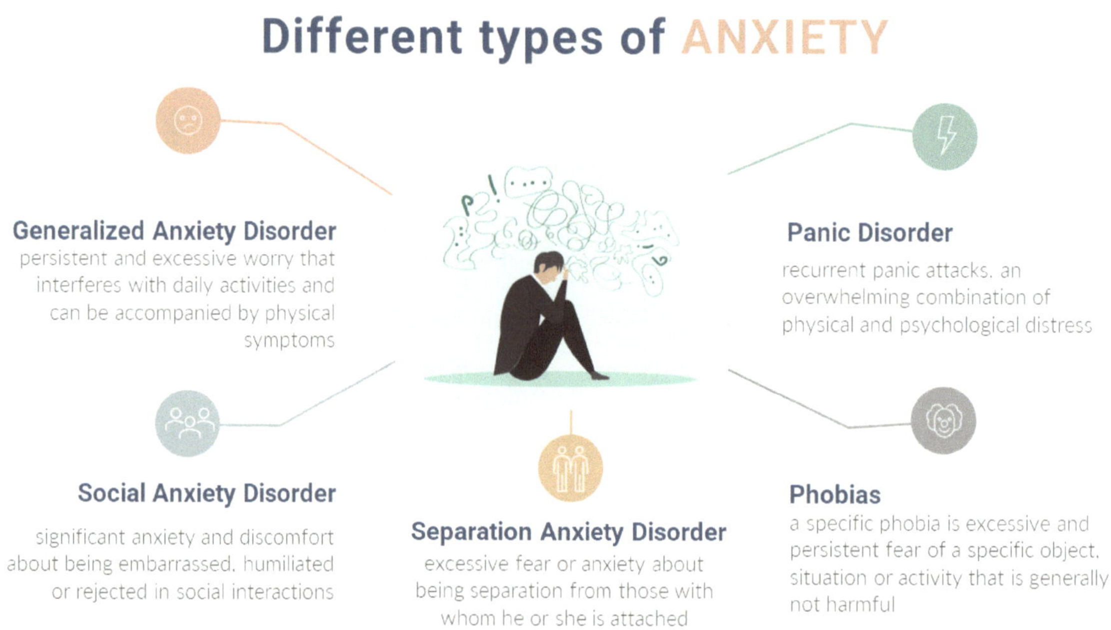

Source: ilovcdtoolkit.org/anxiety-depression

The disturbance persists for at least four weeks in children and adolescents and typically six months or more in adults, causing significant distress or impairment. The diagnosis recognizes that separation anxiety represents normal development at certain ages, becoming pathological when excessive for the developmental stage, persistent, and impairing.

Selective Mutism

Selective Mutism involves consistent failure to speak in specific social situations where speaking is expected, despite speaking in other situations. The disturbance interferes with educational or occupational achievement or social communication, lasts at least one month (not limited to the first month of school), and is not attributable to lack of knowledge or comfort with the language or to another communication disorder.

This disorder typically manifests in early childhood and is considered an anxiety disorder because the failure to speak relates to anxiety about social situations. Children with selective mutism typically speak freely at home with family but become mute in school or public settings. The condition often accompanies social anxiety disorder.

Depressive Disorders

Depressive disorders are characterized by a sad, empty, or irritable mood accompanied by somatic and cognitive changes significantly affecting functioning. They differ based on duration, timing, and presumed etiology.

Major Depressive Disorder (MDD)

Major Depressive Disorder requires at least one major depressive episode. A major depressive episode consists of five or more of nine symptoms present during the same two-week period, representing a change from previous functioning, with at least one symptom being either depressed mood or loss of interest or pleasure (anhedonia).

The nine symptoms are:

1. Depressed mood most of the day, nearly every day (in children and adolescents, can be irritable mood)
2. Markedly diminished interest or pleasure in all or almost all activities most of the day, nearly every day
3. Significant weight loss when not dieting or weight gain, or a decrease or increase in appetite nearly every day (in children, failure to make expected weight gain)
4. Insomnia or hypersomnia nearly every day

5. Psychomotor agitation or retardation nearly every day observable by others
6. Fatigue or loss of energy nearly every day
7. Feelings of worthlessness or excessive or inappropriate guilt nearly every day
8. Diminished ability to think or concentrate, or indecisiveness, nearly every day
9. Recurrent thoughts of death, recurrent suicidal ideation without a specific plan, suicide attempt, or specific plan for committing suicide

The symptoms cause clinically significant distress or impairment, are not attributable to substances or medical conditions, have never been accompanied by a manic or hypomanic episode (which would indicate bipolar disorder), and are not better explained by schizophrenia spectrum or other psychotic disorders.

MDD is further characterized by numerous specifiers indicating features that may guide treatment or predict course:

- **Severity specifiers**: Mild, moderate, severe (based on symptom number, intensity, and impairment level). A "with psychotic features" specifier indicates the presence of delusions or hallucinations, which may be mood-congruent (consistent with depressive themes) or mood-incongruent.
- **Course specifiers**: In partial remission (previously met full criteria, now only some symptoms present) or in full remission (no significant symptoms for at least two months).

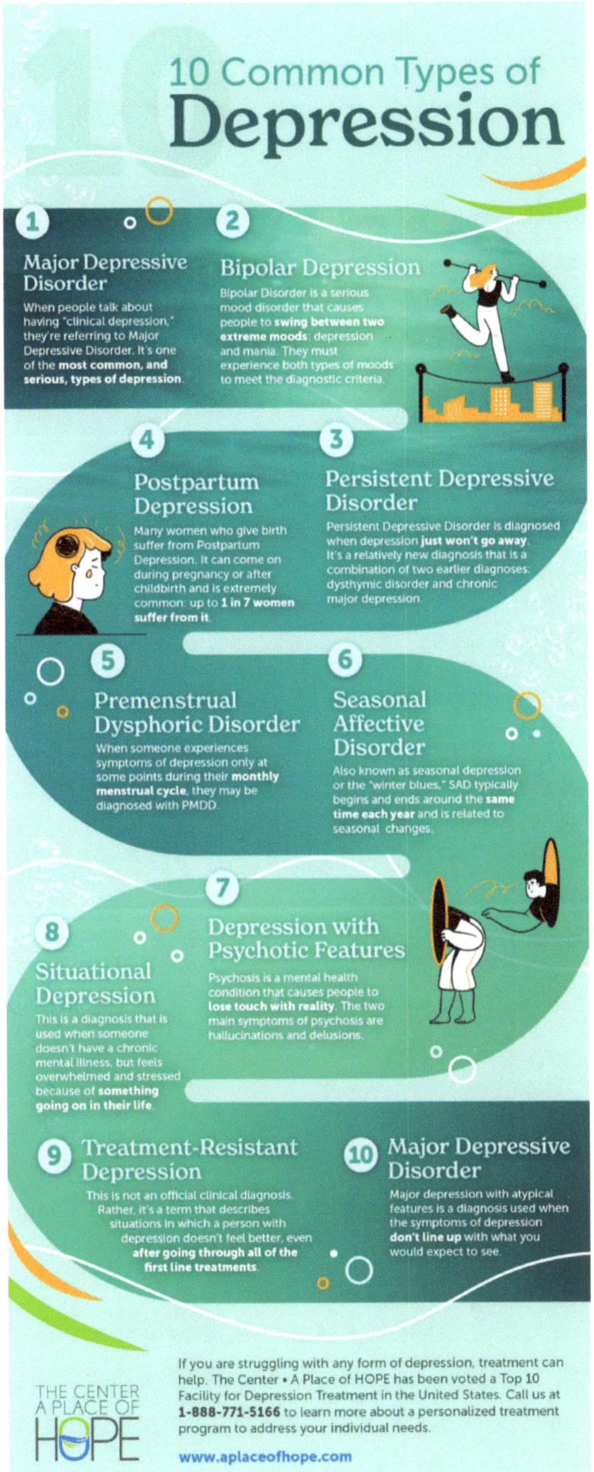
10 Common Types of
Depression
1
Major Depressive Disorder
When people talk about having "clinical depression," they're referring to Major Depressive Disorder. It's one of the most common, and serious, types of depression.
2
Bipolar Depression
Bipolar Disorder is a serious mood disorder that causes people to swing between two extreme moods: depression and mania. They must experience both types of moods to meet the diagnostic criteria.
3
Persistent Depressive Disorder
Persistent Depressive Disorder is diagnosed when depression just won't go away. It's a relatively new diagnosis that is a combination of two earlier diagnoses: dysthymic disorder and chronic major depression.
4
Postpartum Depression
Many women who give birth suffer from Postpartum Depression. It can come on during pregnancy or after childbirth and is extremely common: up to 1 in 7 women suffer from it.
5
Premenstrual Dysphoric Disorder
When someone experiences symptoms of depression only at some points during their monthly menstrual cycle, they may be diagnosed with PMDD.
6
Seasonal Affective Disorder
Also known as seasonal depression or the "winter blues," SAD typically begins and ends around the same time each year and is related to seasonal changes.
7
Depression with Psychotic Features
Psychosis is a mental health condition that causes people to lose touch with reality. The two main symptoms of psychosis are hallucinations and delusions.
8
Situational Depression
This is a diagnosis that is used when someone doesn't have a chronic mental illness, but feels overwhelmed and stressed because of something going on in their life.
9
Treatment-Resistant Depression
This is not an official clinical diagnosis. Rather, it's a term that describes situations in which a person with depression doesn't feel better, even after going through all of the first line treatments.
10
Major Depressive Disorder
Major depression with atypical features is a diagnosis used when the symptoms of depression don't line up with what you would expect to see.
THE CENTER A PLACE OF HOPE
If you are struggling with any form of depression, treatment can help. The Center • A Place of HOPE has been voted a Top 10 Facility for Depression Treatment in the United States. Call us at 1-888-771-5166 to learn more about a personalized treatment program to address your individual needs.
www.aplaceofhope.com

Additional specifiers:

- **With anxious distress**: Feeling keyed up or tense, restlessness, difficulty concentrating due to worry, fear that something awful may happen, or fear of losing control
- **With mixed features**: At least three manic/hypomanic symptoms present but not meeting full criteria for a manic episode
- **With melancholic features**: Anhedonia plus three of: distinct quality of depressed mood, depression worse in morning, early morning awakening, marked psychomotor changes, significant anorexia or weight loss, excessive guilt
- **With atypical features**: Mood reactivity (mood brightens in response to positive events) plus two of: significant weight gain or increased appetite, hypersomnia, leaden paralysis (heavy feeling in limbs), interpersonal rejection sensitivity
- **With mood-congruent psychotic features**: Delusions or hallucinations consistent with depressive themes (guilt, deserved punishment, nihilism, disease)
- **With mood-incongruent psychotic features**: Delusions or hallucinations not consistent with depressive themes
- **With catatonia**: Presence of catatonic features (motoric immobility, excessive motor activity, mutism, peculiar movements)
- **With peripartum onset**: Onset during pregnancy or within four weeks postpartum
- **With seasonal pattern**: Regular temporal relationship between episode onset and particular time of year (typically fall/winter), with remissions also seasonally patterned

These specifiers recognize MDD heterogeneity and guide treatment selection. For example, atypical features suggest preferential response to certain antidepressants, while psychotic features necessitate combination treatment with antipsychotics or electroconvulsive therapy consideration.

Persistent Depressive Disorder (Dysthymia)

Persistent Depressive Disorder represents chronic depression, requiring depressed mood for most of the day, more days than not, for at least two years (one year in children/adolescents). During this period, at least two of six symptoms must be present: poor appetite or overeating, insomnia or hypersomnia, low energy or fatigue, low self-esteem, poor concentration or difficulty making decisions, and feelings of hopelessness.

The individual has never been without symptoms for more than two months during the two-year period. Criteria for major depressive episode may be continuously present for two years, in which case both persistent depressive disorder and major depressive disorder diagnoses apply. The distinction from MDD lies in chronicity rather than severity—persistent depressive disorder can range from mild to severe but must be persistent.

This diagnosis consolidates what DSM-IV classified separately as chronic major depression and dysthymic disorder, recognizing that the distinction was often arbitrary and that chronic depression, regardless of whether it meets full major depressive episode criteria continuously, represents a clinically meaningful condition requiring treatment.

Specifiers include: with anxious distress; with mixed features; with melancholic features; with atypical features; with mood-congruent psychotic features; with mood-incongruent psychotic features; with peripartum onset; current severity: mild, moderate, severe; early onset: before age 21; late onset: age 21 or older, with pure dysthymic syndrome: full criteria for a major depressive episode have not been met in the preceding two years; with persistent major depressive episode: full major depressive episode criteria have been met throughout the preceding two-year period; with intermittent major depressive episodes, with current episode: current major depressive episode but episodes have not persisted continuously over two years; with intermittent major depressive episodes, without current episode: no current major depressive episode but history of episodes during the two-year dysthymic period

Disruptive Mood Dysregulation Disorder (DMDD)

Disruptive Mood Dysregulation Disorder was introduced in DSM-5 to address concerns about overdiagnosis of bipolar disorder in children exhibiting severe irritability and temper outbursts. The disorder is diagnosed in children aged 6-18 years and involves severe recurrent temper outbursts manifested verbally or behaviorally that are grossly out of proportion to the situation and developmental level, occurring on average three or more times per week.

Between outbursts, mood is persistently irritable or angry most of the day, nearly every day, and observable by others (parents, teachers, peers). Symptoms have been present for 12 or more months, with no period lasting three or more consecutive months without all symptoms. Symptoms are present in at least two settings (e.g., home, school, with peers) and are severe in at least one of these settings.

The diagnosis cannot be made before age 6 or after age 18, cannot coexist with oppositional defiant disorder, intermittent explosive disorder, or bipolar disorder (though it can coexist with MDD, ADHD, conduct disorder, and substance use disorders), and symptoms are not better explained by another mental disorder or physiological effects of substances or medical conditions.

DMDD remains somewhat controversial, with critics arguing it pathologizes normal childhood irritability and supporters contending it prevents inappropriate bipolar disorder diagnosis and treatment. Longitudinally, children with DMDD appear at elevated risk for unipolar depression and anxiety disorders rather than bipolar disorder.

Premenstrual Dysphoric Disorder (PMDD)

Premenstrual Dysphoric Disorder involves a pattern of mood symptoms occurring during the premenstrual phase of menstrual cycles. In the majority of cycles during the past year, at least five of eleven symptoms must be present in the week before menses onset, improve within a few days after menses onset, and become minimal or absent in the week post-menses.

At least one symptom must be from the following four: marked affective lability (mood swings), marked irritability or anger, or increased interpersonal conflicts, marked depressed mood or hopelessness or self-deprecating thoughts, and marked anxiety or tension or feelings of being keyed up or on edge.

Additional symptoms include decreased interest in activities, difficulty concentrating, lethargy or marked lack of energy, significant changes in appetite, hypersomnia or insomnia, a sense of being overwhelmed or out of control, and physical symptoms (such as breast tenderness, joint or muscle pain, bloating, or weight gain). Symptoms cause clinically significant distress or interference with work, school, social activities, or relationships.

The diagnosis requires prospective daily ratings during at least two symptomatic cycles to confirm the temporal pattern. PMDD is distinguished from premenstrual syndrome (PMS) by severity and functional impairment. The disorder reflects mood sensitivity to normal hormonal fluctuations rather than hormonal abnormalities per se. Neurobiological mechanisms involve interactions between ovarian steroids and central nervous system neurotransmitter systems, particularly serotonergic function.

Depressive Disorder Due to Another Medical Condition

This diagnosis applies when a depressive syndrome is judged to be the direct pathophysiological consequence of a medical condition. The disturbance must cause clinically significant distress or impairment and not occur exclusively during delirium. Evidence from history, physical examination, or laboratory findings must indicate that the disturbance is etiologically related to the medical condition through a physiological mechanism.

Medical conditions commonly associated with secondary depression include:

- **Neurological**: borderline disorders
- **Endocrine**: Hypothyroidism, hyperthyroidism, Cushing's syndrome, Addison's disease
- **Metabolic**: Vitamin B12 deficiency, folate deficiency, hypercalcemia, hepatic encephalopathy
- **Infectious**: HIV/AIDS, neurosyphilis, Lyme disease
- **Autoimmune**: Systemic lupus erythematosus, multiple sclerosis
- **Malignancies**: Pancreatic cancer, brain tumors

Distinguishing primary depression from depression secondary to medical conditions can be challenging, as many medical conditions increase depression risk through both physiological mechanisms and psychosocial stress of chronic illness. The diagnosis requires evidence that the medical condition directly causes depressive symptoms through known pathophysiological mechanisms.

Substance/Medication-Induced Depressive Disorder

This disorder involves a prominent and persistent depressed mood or anhedonia predominating the clinical picture, developing during or soon after substance intoxication or withdrawal, or after medication exposure, with the substance or medication capable of producing the symptoms. The disturbance causes significant distress or impairment and is not better explained by independent depressive disorder.

Numerous substances can induce depression:

- **Alcohol**: Particularly during withdrawal
- **Sedatives, hypnotics, anxiolytics**: During intoxication or withdrawal
- **Stimulants**: Particularly during withdrawal (cocaine, amphetamines)
- **Opioids**: During intoxication or withdrawal
- **Cannabis**: Some individuals experience depressive symptoms

Medications associated with depression include:

- **Corticosteroids**: Particularly with high doses or chronic use
- **Interferon**: Used in hepatitis C treatment
- **Beta-blockers**: Some cardiovascular medications
- **Isotretinoin**: Acne medication
- **Hormonal contraceptives**: In susceptible individuals

The diagnosis requires temporal association between substance/medication exposure and symptom onset and improvement following substance discontinuation, though symptoms may persist for weeks depending on the substance's half-life and withdrawal course.

Other Specified Depressive Disorder and Unspecified Depressive Disorder

These residual categories apply when depressive symptoms cause clinically significant distress or impairment but do not meet full criteria for any specific depressive disorder. "Other specified" is used when the clinician chooses to communicate that the specific reason criteria are not met. Examples include:

- **Recurrent brief depression**: Depressive episodes lasting 2-13 days, occurring at least once monthly for 12 months, meeting symptom criteria for major depressive episode except duration
- **Short-duration depressive episode**: Depressive period lasting 4-13 days meeting all symptom criteria for major depressive episode except the two-week duration requirement
- **Depressive episode with insufficient symptoms**: Depressed mood and at least one other depressive symptom lasting at least two weeks but not meeting the five-symptom threshold

"Unspecified depressive disorder" is used when the clinician chooses not to specify the reason, the criteria are not met, or when insufficient information precludes a more specific diagnosis (such as in emergency settings).

Chapter 5

Clinical Manifestations

Stress, anxiety, and depression are related but distinct emotional and physiological states that can significantly interfere with daily functioning. They can share several symptoms—such as sleep changes, concentration difficulties, irritability, and physical complaints—making it challenging to differentiate them clinically. However, their underlying triggers, emotional tone, and duration tend to differ. Stress typically arises as a direct response to external challenges or demands and often resolves once the situation improves. Anxiety is characterized by excessive worry and fear about potential future threats, even when no immediate danger exists. Depression, in contrast, is marked by a persistent loss of interest, low mood, and reduced energy that affect the ability to experience pleasure or motivation. Understanding these differences is crucial for accurate diagnosis and appropriate treatment, as each condition follows its own course and requires tailored interventions.

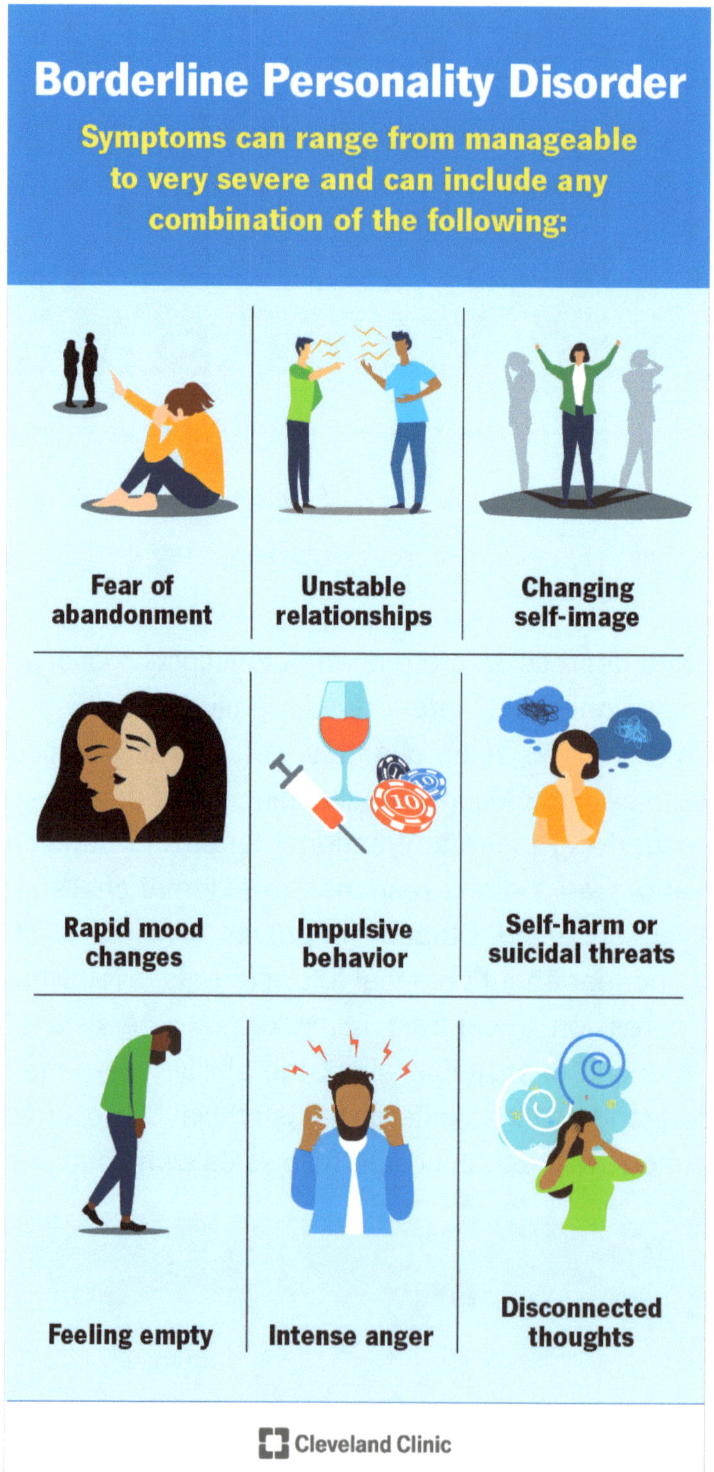
Borderline Personality Disorder
Symptoms can range from manageable to very severe and can include any combination of the following:
Fear of abandonment
Unstable relationships
Changing self-image
Rapid mood changes
Impulsive behavior
10
Self-harm or suicidal threats
Feeling empty
Intense anger
Disconnected thoughts
Cleveland Clinic

Clinical Manifestations of Stress

Stress is a biopsychosocial response to real or perceived threats. Manifestations depend on duration (acute vs chronic) and an individual's coping capacity.

A. Physical manifestations

- Headache, dizziness
- Muscle tension (neck, shoulders, back pain)
- Palpitations, increased heart rate, and blood pressure
- Gastrointestinal issues: nausea, abdominal pain, diarrhea, or constipation
- Fatigue, sleep disturbance (insomnia, restless sleep)
- Excessive sweating, trembling
- Worsening of pre-existing medical conditions (e.g., eczema, hypertension)

B. Cognitive manifestations

- Difficulty concentrating, distractibility
- Memory lapses
- Intrusive thoughts about the stressor
- Overthinking, indecisiveness

C. Emotional manifestations

- Irritability, frustration
- Feeling overwhelmed or "on edge"
- Anxiety or fear linked to the stressor
- Reduced tolerance for everyday challenges

D. Behavioral manifestations

- Changes in eating patterns (overeating or reduced appetite)
- Sleep pattern disruptions
- Avoidance of situations related to the stressor
- Increased use of alcohol, caffeine, and smoking
- Social withdrawal or decreased productivity

If symptoms persist after the stressor ends or cause significant impairment, the condition may progress to adjustment disorder or contribute to anxiety/depression.

Clinical Manifestations of Anxiety

Anxiety involves excessive worry and heightens physiological arousal disproportionate to the situation.

A. Physical manifestations

- Rapid heartbeat, chest tightness
- Shortness of breath, hyperventilation
- Trembling, muscle tension
- Gastrointestinal distress (e.g., irritable bowel-like symptoms)
- Dizziness, sweating, dry mouth
- Sleep difficulties due to rumination or fear
- Panic attacks in some disorders (sudden, intense fear, feeling of loss of control)

B. Cognitive manifestations

- Persistent worry, "racing thoughts"
- Catastrophic thinking (anticipating worst outcomes)

- Impaired concentration and attentional shifts to perceived threats
- Derealization or depersonalization may occur in severe panic states

C. Emotional manifestations

- Fear, apprehension, or intense nervousness
- Increased startle response
- Feelings of dread without clear triggers

D. Behavioral manifestations

- Avoidance of feared objects/situations (e.g., social situations, travel)
- Reassurance-seeking
- Restlessness, fidgeting
- Reduced functioning in social/work/school activities

Clinical Manifestations of Depression

Depression is a persistent disturbance of mood and emotional regulation, often affecting cognition and physical health.

A. Emotional manifestations

- Persistent sadness, emptiness, or hopelessness
- Irritability (especially in children/adolescents)
- Anhedonia: loss of interest or pleasure in usual activities
- Low self-esteem, guilt, feelings of worthlessness

B. Cognitive manifestations

- Negative thinking patterns (self-blame, pessimism)
- Difficulty concentrating, slowed thinking

- Impaired memory
- Indecision and reduced motivation
- Suicidal thoughts or preoccupation with death in severe cases

C. Physical (somatic) manifestations

- Fatigue, low energy
- Sleep changes: insomnia or hypersomnia
- Appetite and weight changes (increase or loss)
- Psychomotor changes: agitation or slowing
- Pain without clear medical cause (e.g., headaches, back pain)

D. Behavioral manifestations

- Withdrawal from social interaction
- Decline in occupational or academic performance
- Neglect of personal care
- Reduced speech and movement (in severe episodes)

Key Distinguishing Features

Feature	Stress	Anxiety	Depression
Primary trigger	External stressor	Perceived threat, often vague	Internal negative mood
Time orientation	Usually, present situation	Future-focused worry	Past or internal state
Thought speed	Rapid but situational	Racing, catastrophic	Slowed, pessimistic
Dominant emotion	Tension, overload	Fear, worry	Sadness, emptiness
Typical onset	Linked to events	May be spontaneous	Gradual or episodic
Arousal level	Increased	Increased	Often reduced (but may be agitated)
Sleep	Difficulty falling asleep	Difficulty staying asleep	Early morning awakening or oversleeping

Clinical relevance

- These three conditions frequently co-occur and can exacerbate one another.
- Early identification of symptoms in schools, workplaces, and primary care settings leads to improved outcomes.
- For children (like your son), somatic symptoms, irritability, and behavioral change often dominate the clinical picture rather than verbal expression of distress.

Chapter 6

Diagnosis and Assessment Tools

Stress

Diagnosing stress typically begins with a thorough clinical interview focused on recent life events, perceived burdens, coping resources, and physical symptoms. Because stress is a natural adaptive response rather than a formal psychiatric disorder, diagnosis centers on identifying when the response becomes excessive, persistent, or harmful to health. Also evaluated the cognitive and emotional impact of stress, such as irritability, worry, reduced concentration, and feelings of being overwhelmed. Red flags include deteriorating work or academic performance, social withdrawal, and persistent physical complaints. In addition to psychological screening instruments, the further assessment includes behavioral coping strategies, including avoidance patterns, substance use, and changes in eating or sleeping routines. Maladaptive coping—such as increased alcohol consumption, emotional withdrawal, or compulsive behavior—can indicate that stress is progressing toward more severe mental health consequences. Identifying protective factors and resilience (e.g., social support, problem-solving skills) is also crucial, as these influence both prognosis and intervention planning.

Lastly, diagnosis involves determining whether the stress response has led to a secondary clinical condition. Chronic or unmanaged stress is a major risk factor for adjustment disorder (as defined in DSM-5/ICD-11), generalized anxiety, and depressive episodes, as well as somatic conditions such as hypertension, tension headaches, and gastrointestinal disorders. Early recognition through structured assessment allows timely intervention, reducing the likelihood of progression to a diagnosable mental health disorder or significant medical complication.

Physiological assessment is relevant because stress activates the autonomic nervous system and the hypothalamic-pituitary-adrenal (HPA) axis. The other parameters could also be monitored, such as blood pressure, sleep patterns, headache frequency, or gastrointestinal disturbances. Laboratory measures, such as cortisol levels, can support the diagnosis of stress-related conditions but are not diagnostic alone.

Structured tools help quantify stress severity. Common instruments include the Perceived Stress Scale (PSS), Holmes and Rahe Stress Inventory, Cohen's Stress Questionnaire, and Job Stress Surveys. These enable tracking over time and evaluating the effectiveness of interventions.

Diagnosis also requires differentiation from anxiety or depressive disorders. Stress is more directly linked to identifiable external factors, and symptoms typically decrease when the stressor abates. Screening ensures that persistent emotional disturbance does not develop into a clinical disorder.

Anxiety

Anxiety disorders are diagnosed using standardized criteria from DSM-5 or ICD-11, focusing on excessive fear and worry that are disproportionate to actual threats and impair functioning. A clinical interview explores triggers, duration (typically ≥6 months for generalized anxiety disorder), and avoidance behaviors.

Somatic symptoms—palpitations, sweating, shortness of breath, dizziness, muscle tension, stomach discomfort—are evaluated, as they reflect inappropriate physiological activation in non-dangerous contexts. Persistent anticipatory worry about everyday scenarios is characteristic. Assessment also explores avoidance behaviors and their impact on independence and daily functioning, since avoiding feared situations strengthens anxiety over time and reduces quality of life. Diagnostic interviews assess whether worry extends across multiple life domains (such as school, work, health, and social interactions) or is tied to specific triggers. Cognitive patterns—like catastrophic thinking and heightened sensitivity to uncertainty—are examined to better understand the nature and severity of anxiety.

Screening also checks for co-occurring mental health conditions such as depression, obsessive–compulsive symptoms, or trauma-related disorders, which frequently overlap with anxiety presentations. Possible physical contributors such as thyroid imbalance, stimulant use, cardiac irregularities, or respiratory problems should also be excluded. Early recognition and differentiation support the prevention of chronic anxiety and long-term impairment.

Diagnostic tools help differentiate types of anxiety disorders, such as generalized anxiety disorder, panic disorder, social anxiety disorder, phobias, and separation anxiety. Whether the anxiety is situational or generalized across contexts could also be screened. Validated scales provide quantitative measurement. Widely used instruments include the GAD-7 (Generalized Anxiety Disorder-7), the Hamilton Anxiety Rating Scale (HAM-A), the Beck Anxiety Inventory (BAI), and the State-Trait Anxiety Inventory (STAI). These tools support monitoring response to treatment in clinical and research settings.

Rule-outs are essential: anxiety symptoms may mimic cardiac, endocrine, or respiratory diseases. Evaluation may include thyroid function tests, ECG, and metabolic panels. Comorbid depression is also common and should be screened because it worsens prognosis and influences intervention strategies.

Diagnostic Focus and Assessment Tools for Stress, Anxiety, and Depression.

Feature	Stress	Anxiety	Depression
Diagnostic classification	Not a formal ICD-11/DSM-5 disorder (but symptoms may contribute to adjustment disorders)	Classified as anxiety disorders in DSM-5 / ICD-11 (e.g., GAD, panic disorder, phobias)	Classified as depressive disorders in DSM-5 / ICD-11 (e.g., Major Depressive Disorder)
Core focus of diagnosis	Response to identifiable external stressor; severity and impact on daily functioning	Excessive fear and worry, often disproportionate to risk; anticipation of future threats	Persistent low mood and/or loss of pleasure affecting functioning ≥2 weeks
Typical symptoms emphasized	Irritability, tension, fatigue, sleep disruption, somatic complaints	Autonomic hyperarousal (e.g., palpitations, shortness of breath), restlessness, avoidance behaviors	Sleep/appetite changes, low energy, guilt, psychomotor changes, suicidal ideation
Diagnostic timeframe	Variable; usually linked to duration of stressor	≥6 months for generalized anxiety disorder (per DSM-5)	≥2 weeks for major depression

Feature	Stress	Anxiety	Depression
Main psychological tools used	Perceived Stress Scale (PSS), Holmes & Rahe Inventory, Job Stress Survey	GAD-7, HAM-A, BAI, STAI	PHQ-9, BDI, HAM-D, MADRS, EPDS (postnatal)
Medical/ biological assessment	Sometimes cortisol and autonomic measures (supporting but not diagnostic)	May require cardiac/endocrine/respiratory rule-outs	Rule-out thyroid disease, anemia, vitamin deficiencies; assess suicide risk
Differential diagnosis considerations	Differentiate situational stress from anxiety and depressive disorders	Exclude physical causes and bipolar depression; assess if fear is situational or generalized	Differentiate unipolar from bipolar disorders; check for comorbid anxiety
Common comorbidities	Anxiety, depression, sleep disorders	Depression, substance use, stress-related disorders	Anxiety disorders, cognitive impairment in severe/recurrent depression

Depression

Depression diagnosis relies on identifying persistent low mood or loss of interest/pleasure, along with additional symptoms such as sleep changes, appetite disturbances, low energy, feelings of guilt, psychomotor changes, and suicidal thoughts. Symptoms must last at least two weeks and cause significant impairment to meet DSM-5/ICD-11 criteria for a depressive disorder.

Clinical interviews examine the onset, course, precipitating factors, and functioning across personal, academic, social, and occupational areas. Mood congruence, level of insight, and presence of cognitive distortions (hopelessness, negative self-beliefs) are carefully assessed.

Assessment also focuses on differentiating unipolar depression from bipolar disorder, because treatment strategies differ fundamentally. Screening for past hypomanic or manic episodes is essential, particularly before prescribing antidepressants.

Multiple validated screening and severity tools are used in clinical care and research. Common examples include the PHQ-9 (Patient Health Questionnaire-9), Hamilton Depression Rating Scale (HAM-D), Beck Depression Inventory (BDI), Montgomery-Åsberg Depression Rating Scale (MADRS), and Edinburgh Postnatal Depression Scale (EPDS), which are particularly relevant in perinatal contexts.

Because depression may have biological contributors, medical evaluation is sometimes indicated—particularly to rule out anemia, thyroid dysfunction, vitamin deficiencies, and neurological illness. Assessment of suicide risk is a core part of every evaluation and requires immediate intervention when positive. A thorough diagnostic evaluation includes assessment of suicidal thoughts or self-harm behaviors, along with identification of both protective and risk factors. A lifetime history of mood symptoms, traumatic experiences, and family patterns of mood disorders helps determine vulnerability and severity. Cognitive themes—such as hopelessness, excessive guilt, and negative self-beliefs—serve as important severity indicators and require close monitoring.

It is also essential to distinguish depressive symptoms from other conditions that may appear similar, such as grief reactions, physical illness, vitamin or thyroid disorders, or substance-related mood changes. Some individuals—including adolescents, men, and older adults—may show predominantly physical or behavioral symptoms rather than verbalizing sadness. Accurate diagnostic distinction ensures proper treatment selection, improves recovery outcomes, and reduces the risk of relapse.

Chapter 7

Neurobiology and solutions of BPDs

Neurobiological Aspects of Stress

Stress triggers a coordinated response involving the central nervous system and the endocrine system, primarily through the activation of the hypothalamic-pituitary-adrenal (HPA) axis. When a stressor is perceived, the hypothalamus releases corticotropin-releasing hormone (CRH), which stimulates the pituitary to secrete adrenocorticotropic hormone (ACTH). ACTH, in turn, prompts the adrenal glands to release cortisol. This hormonal cascade mobilizes energy resources, enhances alertness, and prepares the body to respond to environmental challenges.

The amygdala, a key structure in emotional processing, detects potential threats and initiates the stress response. Activation of the amygdala enhances vigilance, emotional arousal, and memory encoding for emotionally salient events. Simultaneously, the hippocampus provides contextual information, helping to regulate the intensity of the stress response by evaluating the environment and past experiences. Dysregulation in these areas can amplify stress perception, making minor stressors trigger disproportionately intense physiological and emotional responses. When an individual encounters a stressor, the amygdala rapidly evaluates the situation's threat level through both subcortical (thalamo-amygdala) and cortical (thalamo-cortico-amygdala) pathways. The amygdala then activates two major stress response systems: the rapid sympathetic-adrenal-medullary (SAM) axis, which is mediated through projections to brainstem autonomic centers, and the slower hypothalamic-pituitary-adrenal (HPA) axis, which is mediated through projections to the hypothalamus.

The prefrontal cortex, particularly the ventromedial and dorsolateral regions, evaluates the stressor cognitively, implementing conscious appraisal processes that determine whether the situation is truly threatening, controllable, or manageable. The prefrontal cortex can inhibit amygdala activation when cognitive evaluation determines that the threat is minimal or controllable, implementing top-down emotion regulation. The hippocampus contributes contextual information, determining whether the current situation resembles past threatening or safe contexts. This contextual processing enables adaptive fear generalization—responding to situations similar to past threats—while preventing maladaptive overgeneralization to safe situations.

Neurotransmitters such as norepinephrine, dopamine, and serotonin are also implicated in stress responses. Norepinephrine enhances vigilance and prepares the body for immediate action, while dopamine modulates motivation and reward pathways. Serotonin influences mood stability and resilience to stress. Imbalances in these neurotransmitter systems can exacerbate emotional sensitivity, leading to persistent stress reactivity and impaired coping with environmental demands.

The hypothalamic paraventricular nucleus responds to amygdalar signals by releasing corticotropin-releasing hormone (CRH) into the hypophyseal portal system. CRH travels to the anterior pituitary, stimulating corticotroph cells to release adrenocorticotropic hormone (ACTH) into systemic circulation. ACTH reaches the adrenal cortex, triggering the synthesis and release of cortisol. This cascade typically peaks 20-30 minutes after the onset of stress. Simultaneously, the locus coeruleus releases norepinephrine throughout the brain, producing widespread arousal, enhanced vigilance, improved sensory processing, and facilitated memory consolidation for the stressful event. The periaqueductal gray coordinates behavioral responses—fight, flight, or freeze—based on the characteristics of the threat.

Chronic stress leads to structural and functional changes in the brain. Prolonged exposure to cortisol can reduce hippocampal volume, impair memory and contextual evaluation, while increasing amygdala excitability, which heightens emotional reactivity. Similarly, chronic stress can alter prefrontal cortical function, reducing executive control and decision-making abilities. These neuroplastic changes offer a biological explanation for why sustained stress can have a profound impact on cognition, emotion, and behavior.

Stress also engages peripheral systems that communicate with the central nervous system. Sympathetic nervous system activation increases heart rate, blood pressure, and energy mobilization, while immune system activity may be altered via inflammatory signaling pathways. This integration of brain, hormonal, and peripheral systems demonstrates that stress is a comprehensive physiological and neurobiological phenomenon, affecting cognition, emotion, and body-wide homeostasis.

Neurobiological Aspects of Anxiety

Anxiety involves hyperactivation of brain circuits responsible for threat detection and emotional processing. The amygdala plays a central role in this process, rapidly identifying potential dangers and triggering autonomic and behavioral responses. Heightened amygdala activity contributes to exaggerated vigilance and anticipatory worry, even in the absence of immediate threats. This overactivation creates the characteristic sense of tension and hyperarousal observed in anxiety. The amygdala demonstrates heightened reactivity across anxiety disorders, showing exaggerated responses to threatening stimuli and, critically, to ambiguous or even neutral stimuli. This hyperreactivity reflects a lowered threshold for threat detection, causing the individual to perceive danger in situations that are objectively safe. In generalized anxiety disorder, the amygdala shows heightened baseline activity and increased responses to uncertainty and ambiguity. This hyperactivity correlates with worry severity and maintains the chronic anxious state characteristic of GAD. The amygdala's increased functional connectivity with the insula may amplify awareness of anxiety-related bodily sensations.

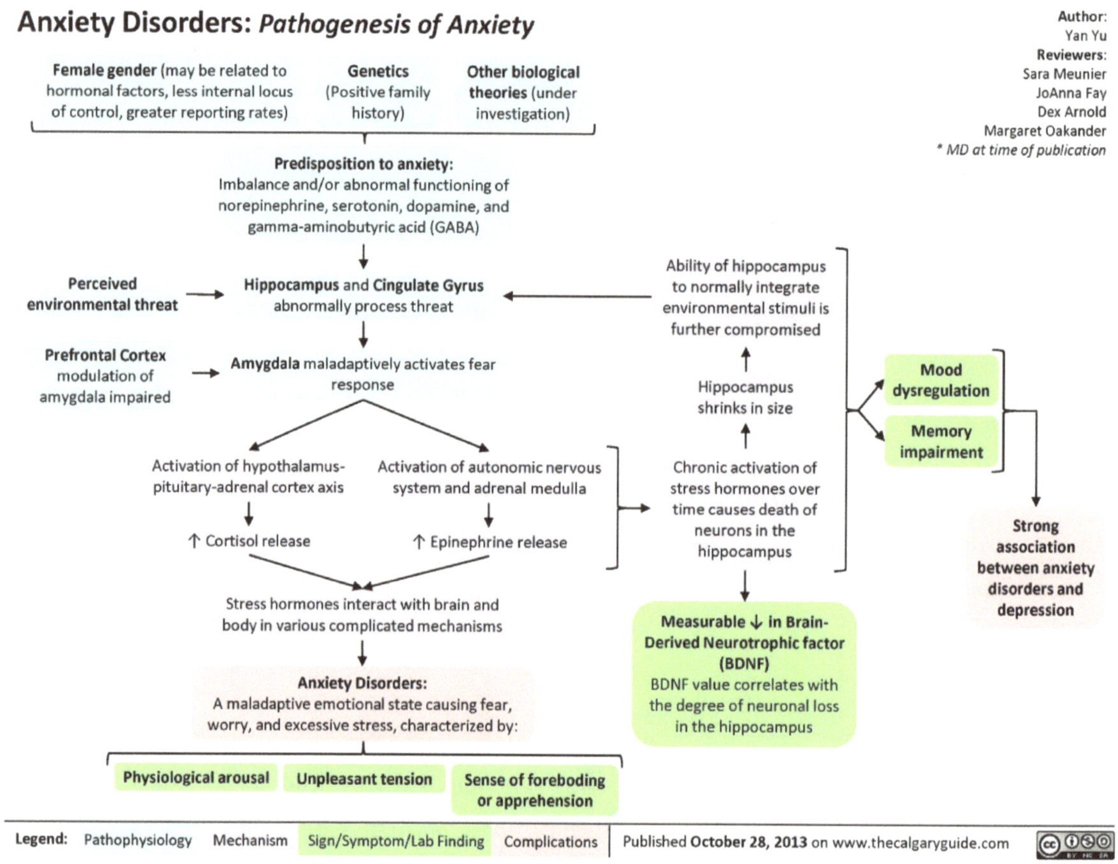

In panic disorder, the amygdala shows heightened responses to interoceptive stimuli—bodily sensations such as increased heart rate, breathlessness, or dizziness. This interoceptive hypersensitivity may trigger panic attacks when normal physiological variations are misinterpreted as catastrophic. The amygdala's connections with the periaqueductal gray may mediate the sudden surge of fear and defensive physiology characteristic of panic.

The prefrontal cortex (PFC) plays a modulatory role in anxiety, particularly the medial and dorsolateral regions, which assess risk and implement cognitive control. Impairment in PFC functioning can reduce its ability to inhibit excessive amygdala responses, leading to persistent anxious thoughts and overestimation of threat. This imbalance between bottom-up emotional signals and top-down cognitive regulation is central to understanding pathological anxiety. Reduced prefrontal cortex function represents a common feature across anxiety disorders, though the specific prefrontal regions affected vary somewhat. The ventromedial prefrontal cortex (vmPFC), crucial for extinction learning and inhibition of fear responses in safe contexts, shows reduced activation and impaired functional connectivity with the amygdala.

This vmPFC dysfunction manifests as difficulty learning that previously feared situations are now safe, causing anxiety to persist even after repeated exposure to evidence of safety. Successful cognitive-behavioral therapy for anxiety disorders increases vmPFC activation and strengthens vmPFC-amygdala functional connectivity, suggesting that therapeutic gains involve restoring this regulatory capacity. The dorsolateral prefrontal cortex exhibits reduced engagement during tasks that require attention control and cognitive reappraisal. This impairment contributes to difficulty disengaging attention from threats and implementing cognitive strategies to reduce anxiety. In GAD, reduced dlPFC function correlates with difficulty controlling worry despite recognition that the worry is excessive. The anterior cingulate cortex demonstrates altered function across anxiety disorders. The dorsal ACC shows heightened activity in response to errors, conflicts, and uncertainty, potentially reflecting excessive performance monitoring and hypervigilance for mistakes. This ACC hyperactivity may underlie the perfectionism, self-criticism, and anticipatory anxiety common in anxiety disorders. In social anxiety disorder, the ACC shows exaggerated responses to social performance situations, correlating with fear of negative evaluation. The subgenual anterior cingulate cortex (area 25), which is important for autonomic regulation and emotional processing, exhibits altered connectivity with the amygdala and insula. This dysfunction may contribute to the autonomic symptoms of anxiety—rapid heart rate, sweating, trembling, gastrointestinal distress—and the difficulty regulating these physiological responses.

The hippocampus is involved in contextualizing threats and distinguishing safe from dangerous environments. In anxiety, hippocampal dysfunction can impair this contextual processing, causing individuals to perceive threats in neutral situations. This misattribution contributes to generalized or persistent anxiety and reinforces avoidance behaviors, as the brain interprets benign contexts as potentially harmful. The hippocampus shows both structural and functional alterations in anxiety disorders. Reduced hippocampal volumes have been documented in PTSD, panic disorder, and social anxiety disorder, potentially reflecting stress-induced atrophy or pre-existing vulnerability factors. Functional imaging reveals impaired hippocampal engagement during contextual fear processing and extinction learning. In PTSD specifically, hippocampal dysfunction manifests as difficulty encoding the contextual details of traumatic memories, leading to fragmented, decontextualized trauma memories that intrude into consciousness. The hippocampus fails to adequately inhibit fear responses in safe contexts, contributing to overgeneralization of fear-responding fearfully to situations that merely resemble trauma contexts rather than representing actual danger.

The hippocampus normally supports pattern separation—the ability to distinguish between similar but distinct contexts or experiences. Impaired pattern separation in anxiety disorders leads to overgeneralization, where fear learned in one context spreads to increasingly dissimilar contexts. For example, someone who experiences a panic attack in a grocery store may begin avoiding all stores, then all public spaces, as the fear generalizes. Reduced hippocampal neurogenesis in anxiety states may contribute to these functional deficits. Animal studies indicate that increasing neurogenesis through exercise, environmental enrichment, or antidepressant treatment reduces anxiety-like behaviors and improves pattern separation, suggesting that neurogenesis may protect against anxiety pathology.

Neurotransmitter systems are critical in the modulation of anxiety. Gamma-aminobutyric acid (GABA) exerts inhibitory control over excitatory circuits, reducing neural overactivation. Dysregulation of GABAergic signaling can heighten anxiety and arousal. Similarly, serotonin regulates mood and threat appraisal, while norepinephrine modulates vigilance and stress-related responses. Imbalances in these systems amplify emotional reactivity and physiological arousal.

Chronic anxiety induces structural and functional neural adaptations. Studies show increased amygdala volume and hyperconnectivity with other limbic regions, which may heighten sensitivity to emotional stimuli. Conversely, prefrontal cortical areas may exhibit reduced thickness or connectivity, thereby impairing the cognitive regulation of fear and worry. Such neuroplastic changes reinforce persistent anxiety, making the nervous system more reactive to perceived threats over time.

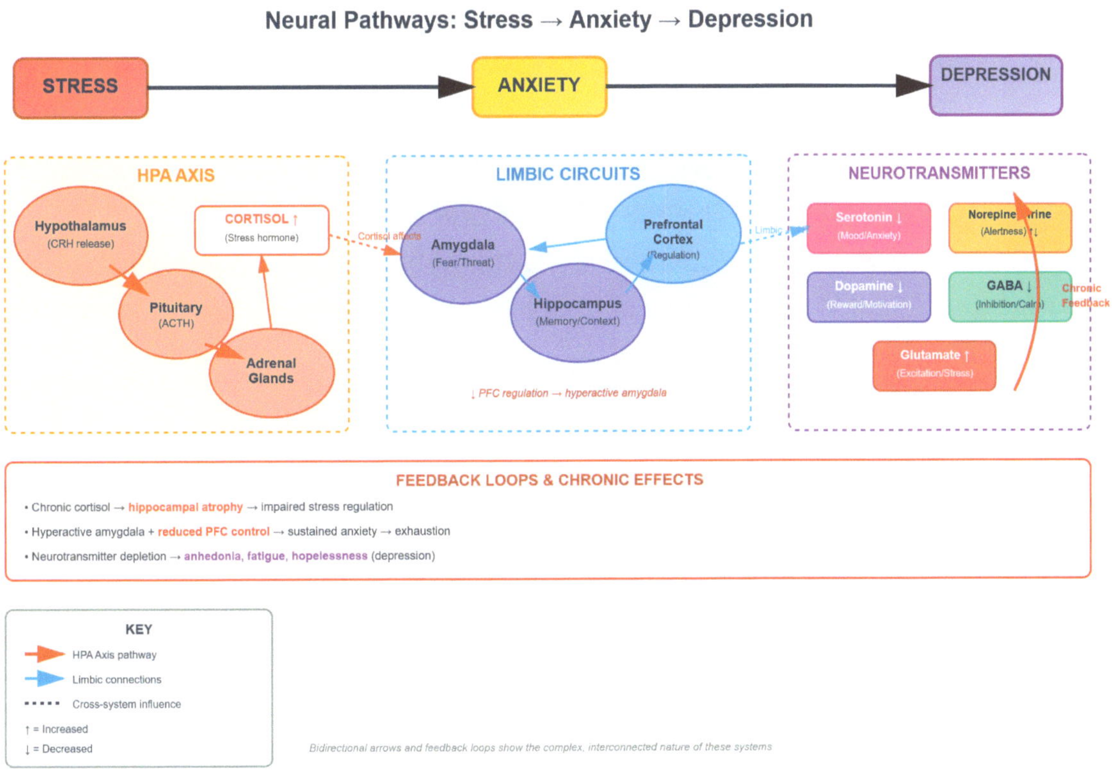

Anxiety also manifests through autonomic and endocrine pathways. Sympathetic nervous system hyperactivity produces rapid heartbeat, sweating, and muscle tension, while HPA axis dysregulation sustains cortisol release, which may contribute to both cognitive and somatic symptoms. Understanding anxiety at the neurobiological level reveals its multi-system nature, linking emotional, cognitive, and physiological processes in a coherent network of threat detection and response.

Neurobiological Aspects of Depression

Depression involves widespread dysregulation across brain regions, neurotransmitter systems, and neuroendocrine pathways. Key brain structures include the prefrontal cortex, which governs executive functioning and emotion regulation;

the amygdala, which processes emotional stimuli; and the hippocampus, which encodes and contextualizes experiences. Functional impairments in these regions contribute to persistent low mood, anhedonia, and cognitive deficits characteristic of depression.

Depression is characterized by reduced activity and diminished volumes in multiple prefrontal regions. The dorsolateral prefrontal cortex shows decreased activation during tasks that require working memory, cognitive control, and executive function, contributing to the concentration difficulties, indecisiveness, and executive dysfunction characteristic of depression. This dlPFC hypofunction impairs cognitive control over emotional processing. Depressed individuals show difficulty implementing cognitive reappraisal strategies to reduce negative emotions, difficulty disengaging from negative information, and difficulty inhibiting rumination. The dlPFC's reduced capacity to downregulate amygdala activity allows unchecked emotional reactivity to negative stimuli.

The ventromedial prefrontal cortex shows complex alterations in depression. Some studies report reduced vmPFC activity, potentially contributing to impaired emotion regulation and difficulty experiencing positive emotions. However, the vmPFC demonstrates increased functional connectivity with the amygdala and subgenual cingulate in depression, possibly reflecting failed attempts at emotion regulation or sustained processing of negative self-referential content. The orbitofrontal cortex, which is involved in processing reward and punishment, exhibits reduced activation to rewarding stimuli and altered value representations. This dysfunction may contribute to anhedonia—the inability to experience pleasure from normally rewarding activities—and to the altered decision-making observed in depression, where depressed individuals often make maladaptive choices reflecting pessimistic outcome expectations.

Structural imaging reveals reduced cortical thickness and gray matter volume in prefrontal regions, particularly with chronic or recurrent depression. These structural changes correlate with illness duration and number of depressive episodes, suggesting progressive effects of depression on brain structure or cumulative effects of stress and glucocorticoid exposure.

The amygdala demonstrates heightened activity in depression, but with characteristics distinct from anxiety disorders. Rather than general threat hypersensitivity, the depressed amygdala shows heightened responses specifically to negative stimuli (sad faces, negative words, loss-related cues) and reduced responses to positive stimuli. This creates a negativity bias, where negative information preferentially captures attention and elicits stronger emotional responses, while positive information is processed less intensely or may be ignored. The amygdala's negative bias contributes to the cognitive distortions characteristic of depression—selective attention to negative aspects of situations, enhanced memory for negative events, and negative interpretation of ambiguous information. This biased processing maintains depressed mood and prevents recognition of positive experiences that might contradict depressive cognitions. In depression, the amygdala shows increased functional connectivity with the subgenual ACC, insula, and medial prefrontal regions involved in self-referential processing. This heightened connectivity may sustain negative affect and link negative emotional responses to self-concept, contributing to feelings of worthlessness and self-criticism. The amygdala also shows reduced habituation to repeated negative stimuli in depression. While healthy individuals show diminishing amygdala responses with repeated exposure to negative images (habituation), depressed individuals maintain strong responses, potentially explaining the sustained negative affect and difficulty moving past negative experiences.

The hippocampus shows some of the most consistent structural changes in depression, with meta-analyses documenting approximately 8-10% volume reductions compared to healthy controls. This atrophy is more pronounced in chronic, recurrent depression and correlates with illness duration and number of depressive episodes. Hippocampal volume loss in depression reflects multiple processes, including chronic glucocorticoid exposure that causes dendritic atrophy and neuronal loss, reduced neurogenesis in the dentate gyrus, decreased brain-derived neurotrophic factor (BDNF) expression, inflammatory processes that damage neurons, and potentially, vascular changes that reduce hippocampal perfusion. Functionally, the hippocampus shows reduced activation during memory encoding in depression, contributing to the memory complaints frequently reported by depressed patients. Depressed individuals particularly show impaired memory for specific autobiographical details and difficulty recalling positive memories in detail, while negative memories remain accessible. This memory bias maintains depression by making negative past experiences readily available while positive memories remain vague. The hippocampus's role in HPA axis negative feedback becomes impaired in depression. Reduced hippocampal glucocorticoid receptor function weakens the hippocampus's ability to terminate stress responses, contributing to HPA axis hyperactivity and sustained hypercortisolemia. This creates a vicious cycle where elevated cortisol further damages the hippocampus, progressively impairing negative feedback. Hippocampal dysfunction also manifests as overgeneralized autobiographical memory-recalling general categorical information ("I have always failed") rather than specific episodic details. This overgeneralization contributes to global negative self-beliefs and difficulty generating specific solutions to problems.

The hypothalamus shows dysregulation across multiple systems in depression. The paraventricular nucleus demonstrates hyperactivity, driving HPA axis overactivation. CRH neurons show increased gene expression, elevated CRH production, and reduced sensitivity to glucocorticoid negative feedback. This results in hypercortisolemia—elevated basal cortisol levels, loss of normal circadian cortisol rhythm, and exaggerated cortisol responses to minor stressors. Approximately 40-50% of depressed patients show abnormal dexamethasone suppression test results, where administration of synthetic glucocorticoid fails to suppress cortisol production as it should. This reflects impaired negative feedback and contributes to chronic glucocorticoid exposure, damaging the hippocampus and other brain regions. The suprachiasmatic nucleus (circadian pacemaker) shows altered function in depression, contributing to disrupted circadian rhythms—disturbed sleep-wake cycles, abnormal cortisol rhythms, altered body temperature regulation, and shifted timing of REM sleep. Depressed individuals often experience early morning awakening, terminal insomnia (waking 2-3 hours before desired wake time and unable to return to sleep), and rapid REM onset. Hypothalamic regulation of appetite becomes disturbed, manifesting as reduced appetite and weight loss in melancholic depression or increased appetite and weight gain in atypical depression. The arcuate nucleus neurons regulating appetite show altered sensitivity to satiety and hunger signals. Hypothalamic regulation of libido becomes impaired, contributing to reduced sexual desire and function commonly reported in depression. This likely involves altered gonadotropin-releasing hormone secretion and reduced responsiveness to sexual cues.

Neurotransmitter systems are central to depressive pathology. Serotonin modulates mood, appetite, and sleep; norepinephrine influences arousal and energy; and dopamine regulates reward and motivation pathways. Dysregulation in these systems contributes to hallmark symptoms such as anhedonia, fatigue, and lack of motivation. These chemical imbalances interact with structural brain changes to sustain depressive states and shape both affective and cognitive experience.

Neuroendocrine dysregulation is a key component of depression. Hyperactivity of the HPA axis leads to elevated cortisol levels, which can impair hippocampal function and reduce neurogenesis, further contributing to cognitive deficits and mood disturbances. Chronic cortisol elevation also affects immune function, linking depression to somatic health outcomes and demonstrating the systemic impact of neurobiological dysregulation.

Chronic depression produces structural and functional neuroplastic changes. Reduced hippocampal volume, altered prefrontal-amygdala connectivity, and impaired reward circuitry are common findings. These alterations reinforce negative cognitive-emotional cycles and contribute to persistent symptoms, highlighting that depression is not merely a temporary mood disturbance but a systemic condition involving multiple interconnected neural networks.

The neurobiological aspects of **Stress, Anxiety, and Depression.**

Aspect	Stress	Anxiety	Depression
Primary Brain Regions	Hypothalamus, Amygdala, Hippocampus, Prefrontal Cortex	Amygdala, Prefrontal Cortex, Hippocampus	Prefrontal Cortex, Amygdala, Hippocampus, Reward Circuitry (Nucleus Accumbens, Ventral Striatum)

Aspect	Stress	Anxiety	Depression
Neuroendocrine Activity	HPA axis activation → CRH → ACTH → Cortisol. Sympathoadrenal medullary (SAM) axis activation (epinephrine/norepinephrine from adrenal medulla)	HPA axis dysregulation; sustained cortisol release in chronic anxiety. Altered insula function (interoceptive awareness)	HPA axis hyperactivity; chronically elevated cortisol affecting hippocampus and cognition. Neuroinflammation and reduced neurogenesis
Neurotransmitters	Norepinephrine, Dopamine, Serotonin; GABA involvement	GABA (inhibitory), Serotonin (mood), Norepinephrine (vigilance)	Serotonin (mood, sleep), Norepinephrine (energy/arousal), Dopamine (motivation, reward)
Amygdala Function	Threat detection, emotional salience	Hyperactive, heightened vigilance and fear processing	Hyperactive, enhanced processing of negative emotional stimuli
Prefrontal Cortex Function	Regulatory control over amygdala; evaluates stressors	Reduced inhibitory control over amygdala → persistent worry	Hypoactive, impaired executive function and cognitive control over negative thoughts

Aspect	Stress	Anxiety	Depression
Hippocampus Function	Contextual evaluation of stressors	Contextual processing of threats; dysfunction leads to generalized anxiety	Impaired memory encoding, reduced volume; limits contextual regulation of mood
Physiological Effects	Sympathetic activation: increased HR, BP, energy mobilization; immune modulation	Autonomic hyperactivity: tachycardia, sweating, muscle tension	Systemic effects: fatigue, sleep disturbances, appetite changes, immune dysregulation
Behavioral Manifestations	Heightened arousal, vigilance, adaptive or maladaptive coping	Hypervigilance, avoidance, repetitive behaviors, anticipatory worry	Withdrawal, anhedonia, reduced motivation, impaired daily functioning
Structural/Plastic Changes	More in chronic stress: hippocampal volume reduction, increased amygdala excitability, PFC dysregulation	Increased amygdala connectivity, reduced PFC thickness, neural sensitization to threats, potential amygdala volume increases	Reduced hippocampal volume, impaired PFC-amygdala connectivity, altered reward circuitry, reduced cortical thickness

Neurotransmitter Overlaps: all three neurotransmitter systems (serotonin, norepinephrine, dopamine) are involved in all three conditions, just with different patterns. HPA Axis in Anxiety: Not all anxiety involves sustained cortisol elevation. Some anxiety disorders show blunted cortisol responses or normal HPA function.

Cellular Changes in Stress, Anxiety, and Depression

The past three decades of neuroscience research have fundamentally transformed understanding of stress-related psychiatric disorders, revealing that conditions once conceptualized primarily as psychological phenomena reflect profound alterations in cellular structure, function, and survival. Major depressive disorder, anxiety disorders, and chronic stress conditions involve measurable changes at the cellular and molecular level, including neuronal atrophy, synaptic remodeling, altered glial function, disrupted neurogenesis, and inflammatory activation. These cellular changes represent the biological substrate underlying the cognitive, emotional, and behavioral symptoms that characterize these disorders.

This cellular pathophysiology perspective has several important implications. First, it validates the biological reality of psychiatric suffering—these are not merely psychological states but conditions involving tangible brain changes. Second, it suggests that effective interventions must address cellular dysfunction, whether through pharmacological agents that modify cellular signaling, psychotherapeutic approaches that promote adaptive neuroplasticity, or emerging strategies directly targeting cellular restoration. Third, it provides a framework for understanding why psychiatric disorders often become chronic and progressive—cellular damage accumulates over time, creating self-perpetuating cycles of dysfunction. Ultimately, it holds promise for novel interventions targeting cellular mechanisms, including approaches that promote neuroplasticity, reduce inflammation, enhance neurotrophic support, and potentially regenerate damaged neural tissue.

Neuronal Structural Changes

Dendritic Atrophy and Spine Loss

Neurons communicate through dendrites—branched processes extending from the cell body that receive input from other neurons via specialized structures called dendritic spines. The complexity of dendritic arbors and the density of spines determine how much information a neuron can integrate and how effectively it can participate in neural circuits. Chronic stress, anxiety disorders, and depression produce dramatic alterations in dendritic structure across multiple brain regions.

Prefrontal cortex dendritic atrophy: Layer II/III and layer V pyramidal neurons in the medial prefrontal cortex show marked dendritic retraction following chronic stress exposure in animal models. The apical dendrites—the primary dendritic branches extending toward the cortical surface—demonstrate reduced length, fewer branches, and simplified branching patterns. This dendritic simplification reduces the neuron's receptive surface area, limiting its capacity to integrate inputs from other cortical regions, the thalamus, and the hippocampus.

Post-mortem studies of individuals who died during depressive episodes reveal similar dendritic pathology in the prefrontal cortex, with reduced dendritic length and complexity compared to psychiatrically healthy individuals. The dorsolateral prefrontal cortex, which is critical for working memory and executive function, exhibits particularly prominent dendritic atrophy, potentially explaining the cognitive symptoms characteristic of depression—difficulty concentrating, impaired decision-making, and reduced cognitive flexibility.

Dendritic spine density also decreases dramatically in the prefrontal cortex with chronic stress and depression. Since each spine represents a potential synaptic connection, spine loss translates directly to reduced synaptic connectivity. This synaptic deficit may represent the structural correlate of prefrontal hypofunction observed in neuroimaging studies. The specific types of spines affected include mushroom spines—mature, stable spines that mediate strong, persistent connections—suggesting that chronic stress disrupts established functional circuits rather than merely preventing formation of new connections.

The mechanisms underlying prefrontal dendritic atrophy involve multiple processes. Chronic glucocorticoid exposure directly affects dendritic structure through genomic and non-genomic mechanisms. Glucocorticoids activate intracellular receptors that translocate to the nucleus and alter gene transcription, downregulating genes supporting dendritic maintenance while upregulating genes promoting dendritic retraction. Glucocorticoids also rapidly affect dendritic structure through membrane-associated receptors that activate signaling cascades affecting the cytoskeleton—the internal scaffolding that maintains dendritic shape.

Reduced brain-derived neurotrophic factor (BDNF) contributes critically to dendritic atrophy. BDNF promotes dendritic growth, enhances synaptic strength, and supports neuronal survival. Chronic stress dramatically reduces BDNF expression in the prefrontal cortex and hippocampus, removing essential neurotrophic support. Without adequate BDNF signaling, dendrites cannot maintain their complex architecture and undergo progressive simplification. Antidepressant medications that increase BDNF can partially reverse stress-induced dendritic atrophy, supporting BDNF's causal role in this pathology.

Excitatory neurotransmission dysregulation also contributes to dendritic damage. Chronic stress increases extracellular glutamate levels while impairing glutamate reuptake by astrocytes. Excessive glutamate activation of NMDA receptors causes calcium influx into neurons, activating enzymes that degrade cytoskeletal proteins and promoting dendritic retraction. This excitotoxic process can progress to neuronal death if sufficiently severe.

Hippocampal dendritic atrophy: The hippocampus shows even more pronounced dendritic changes than the prefrontal cortex in chronic stress and depression. CA3 pyramidal neurons, which possess extensive recurrent connections supporting pattern completion and associative memory, demonstrate dramatic dendritic atrophy following chronic stress. The apical dendrites of CA3 neurons retract by 30 - 40% in animal chronic stress models, with proportional spine loss.

CA1 pyramidal neurons, the primary hippocampal output neurons, similarly show stress-induced dendritic atrophy, though typically less severe than CA3. The dentate gyrus granule cells also exhibit dendritic changes, though these are complicated by the presence of ongoing neurogenesis - stress suppresses production of new granule neurons while also affecting existing neurons' dendritic structure.

Hippocampal dendritic atrophy has profound functional consequences. The hippocampus's role in contextual memory processing depends on its complex internal connectivity, which is disrupted by dendritic simplification. Stress-induced hippocampal dendritic changes correlate with impaired spatial memory, reduced contextual fear conditioning, and impaired ability to distinguish between similar contexts—deficits observed in both animal models and depressed patients.

The hippocampus's vulnerability to stress-induced dendritic changes reflects its exceptionally high glucocorticoid receptor density. While this sensitivity allows the hippocampus to exert negative feedback on the HPA axis during normal stress responses, it renders the structure particularly vulnerable to damage from chronic glucocorticoid elevation. The hippocampus essentially becomes a victim of its own regulatory function.

Inflammatory processes contribute to hippocampal dendritic pathology. Chronic stress activates microglia—the brain's resident immune cells - which release pro-inflammatory cytokines including interleukin-1β (IL-1β), interleukin-6 (IL-6), and tumor necrosis factor-alpha (TNF-α). These cytokines directly affect neuronal function, reducing BDNF production, impairing synaptic plasticity, and promoting dendritic retraction. Anti-inflammatory interventions can partially prevent stress-induced hippocampal dendritic atrophy in animal models, demonstrating inflammation's causal contribution.

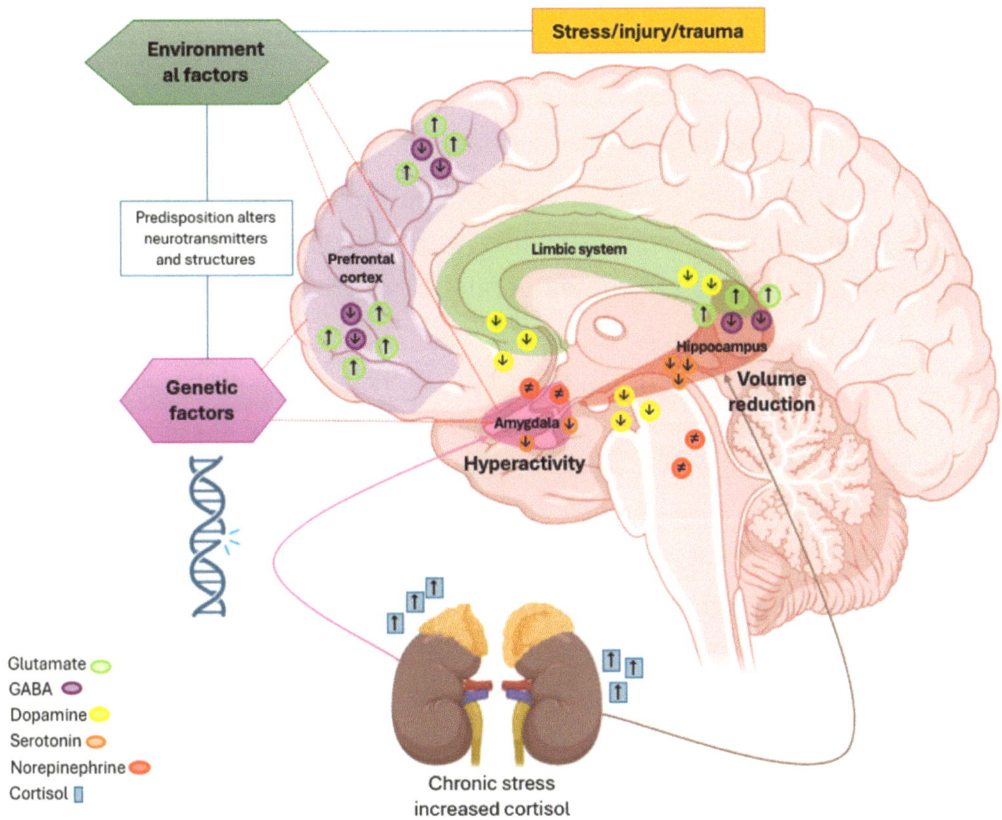

Pathophysiology of anxiety, depression, and stress. Note: Upward arrows imply increase, downward arrows decrease, sign (≠) inhibition of the neurotransmitter.

Source: Estela-Zape JL, Sanclemente-Cardoza V, Noreña-Buitrón LD, Ordoñez-Mora LT. Utilization of Medicinal Plants in Mental Disorders: Neuroplasticity and Neuroprotection in Biomodels. Brain Sciences. 2025; 15(4):366.

Amygdala dendritic changes: Unlike the atrophy observed in the prefrontal cortex and hippocampus, the amygdala shows dendritic growth and increased spine density following chronic stress. Basolateral amygdala principal neurons demonstrate increased dendritic length, enhanced branching complexity, and elevated spine density in chronically stressed animals. This dendritic hypertrophy represents a maladaptive change rather than a healthy adaptation.

Amygdala dendritic growth correlates with heightened anxiety-like behaviors, increased fear conditioning, and impaired fear extinction in animal models. The structural expansion of amygdala neurons appears to enhance the structure's capacity for threat processing while making it more difficult for the prefrontal cortex to exert inhibitory control. The shift in balance—prefrontal atrophy coupled with amygdala hypertrophy—creates a neurobiological state favoring emotional reactivity over cognitive regulation.

The mechanisms driving amygdala dendritic growth differ from those causing atrophy elsewhere. Corticotropin-releasing hormone (CRH), released locally within the amygdala during stress, promotes dendritic growth through CRH type 1 receptors. Glutamatergic neurotransmission enhancement in the amygdala, rather than being toxic as in the hippocampus, promotes activity-dependent dendritic growth. The amygdala's relative paucity of glucocorticoid receptors compared to the hippocampus may protect it from glucocorticoid-induced atrophy while allowing other stress mediators to promote hypertrophy.

This regional specificity of dendritic changes—atrophy in regulatory regions (prefrontal cortex, hippocampus) and hypertrophy in emotional processing regions (amygdala)—creates a neurobiological state biased toward emotional reactivity and away from cognitive control. This cellular imbalance may represent a fundamental substrate of anxiety and depression, explaining why these conditions involve both emotional hyperreactivity and difficulty implementing cognitive coping strategies.

Synaptic Alterations

Beyond dendritic structural changes, stress, anxiety, and depression involve alterations in synapses—the specialized junctions where neurons communicate. Synaptic dysfunction represents a convergent pathway through which multiple pathological processes—altered neurotransmission, reduced neurotrophic support, and inflammatory activation—impair neural circuit function.

Synaptic density reduction: Post-mortem studies of individuals with major depression reveal reduced synaptic density in the prefrontal cortex, with decreases of 20-30% in some cortical layers. The synaptic proteins synaptophysin, synaptotagmin, and complexin - markers of presynaptic terminals—show reduced expression. PSD-95 and other postsynaptic density proteins are similarly decreased, indicating that both sides of the synapse are affected.

This synaptic loss typically occurs without proportional neuronal loss, indicating that neurons survive but with dramatically reduced connectivity. A neuron that loses half its synapses remains alive but functions very differently—it receives less input, integrates information less effectively, and contributes less robustly to circuit function. The cognitive and emotional symptoms of depression may reflect this state of neurons that are alive but poorly connected and functionally compromised.

Synaptic loss correlates with illness duration and severity, suggesting progressive deterioration. First-episode depression shows less synaptic pathology than chronic recurrent depression, and greater symptom severity correlates with more pronounced synaptic deficits. This relationship suggests that each depressive episode may cause additional synaptic damage, lowering the threshold for subsequent episodes—a phenomenon termed "kindling" in psychiatry.

Synaptic plasticity impairment: Beyond static synaptic number, stress and depression impair synaptic plasticity—the capacity of synapses to strengthen or weaken in response to experience. Long-term potentiation (LTP), a cellular mechanism underlying learning and memory in which synapses strengthen following repeated activation, becomes impaired in the hippocampus and prefrontal cortex following chronic stress. Long-term depression (LTD), a complementary mechanism involving synaptic weakening, shows less consistent alterations but may be enhanced in some contexts.

Impaired synaptic plasticity has broad implications beyond memory deficits. Adaptive responses to changing environments require modifying neural circuits through experience-dependent plasticity. Impaired plasticity leaves individuals rigid and unable to update their responses despite changing circumstances. This may explain the cognitive inflexibility characteristic of depression and the difficulty learning that previously feared situations are now safe in anxiety disorders.

The molecular mechanisms underlying plasticity impairment involve multiple systems. BDNF, which promotes both LTP induction and maintenance, becomes reduced. Glutamate receptor expression and function are altered, with reduced AMPA receptor insertion into synapses (critical for LTP) and altered NMDA receptor subunit composition. Calcium signaling cascades that translate synaptic activity into changes in gene expression become disrupted. Epigenetic modifications that regulate plasticity-related gene expression are altered.

Neurotransmitter receptor changes: Chronic alterations in neurotransmitter availability produce compensatory changes in receptor expression and sensitivity. In depression, chronic reductions in serotonin, norepinephrine, and dopamine lead to receptor upregulation—increased receptor density attempting to compensate for reduced neurotransmitter levels. However, this compensation proves inadequate, and receptor function becomes dysregulated.

Serotonin receptors show complex alterations. 5-HT1A receptors, which function as autoreceptors on raphe serotonergic neurons (inhibiting serotonin release) and as postsynaptic receptors in target regions, show reduced sensitivity in depression. This desensitization may reflect chronic stimulation from compensatory mechanisms or may represent a primary defect contributing to depression vulnerability. 5-HT2A receptors show increased density in some brain regions in depression, potentially contributing to anxiety symptoms and sleep disturbance.

Norepinephrine receptors similarly show altered expression. Alpha-2 adrenergic receptors, which serve as autoreceptors inhibiting norepinephrine release, may become hypersensitive in some depressed individuals, excessively suppressing norepinephrine neurotransmission. Beta-adrenergic receptors show region-specific changes in density and coupling to intracellular signaling pathways.

Dopamine receptor alterations in depression particularly affect reward circuits. D2 receptors in the nucleus accumbens, which mediate reward prediction and motivated behavior, show reduced expression and impaired signal transduction. This receptor dysfunction may represent a cellular mechanism for anhedonia—reduced D2 signaling means that rewarding stimuli fail to produce normal dopaminergic responses, subjectively experienced as a lack of pleasure or motivation.

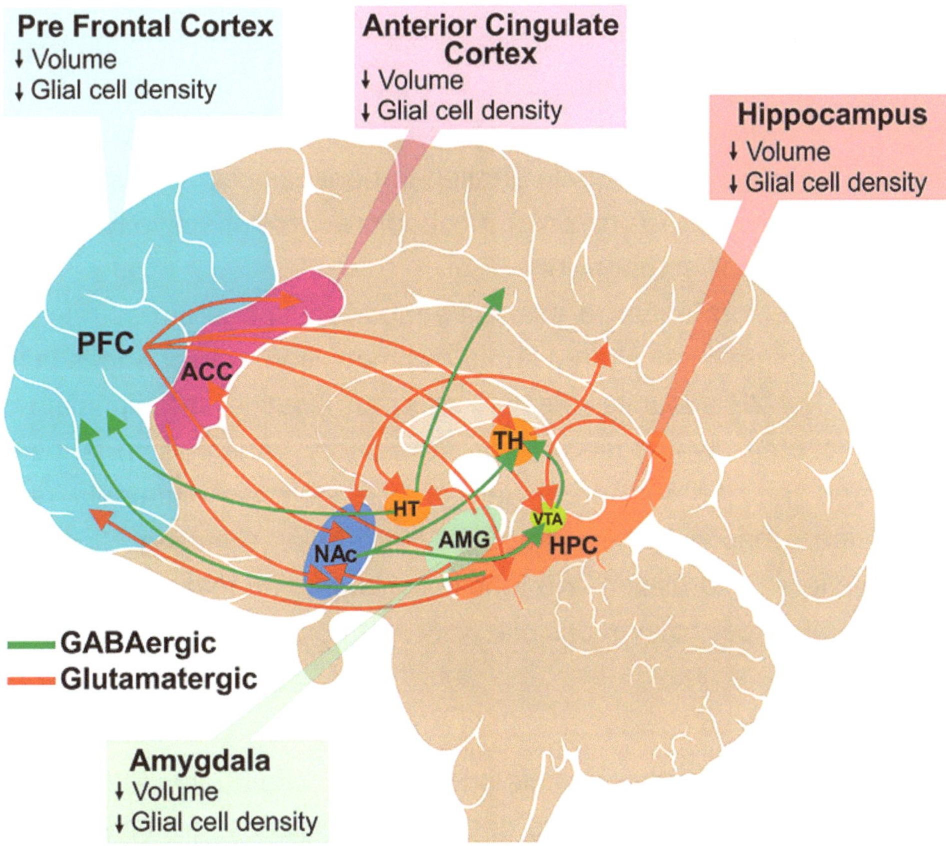

Schematic of glutamatergic and GABAergic projections involved in mood regulation and reward pathway. A subset of several known interconnections among different brain regions are shown. Major glutamatergic projections (red color) arise from the frontal cortex to the anterior cingulate cortex (ACC), thalamus (TH), ventral tegmental area (VTA), hippocampus (HPC) and nucleus accumbens (NAc). Additionally, glutamatergic neurons originate from hippocampus, and innervate into hypothalamus (HT), VTA, NAc and PFC and from amygdala to HT, ACC and NAc. The GABAergic projections (green color) are widely distributed throughout the brain. The major projections that are relevant to this review are from HT to the occipital and parietal cortex, HPC to PFC, and NAc to the thalamus and VTA. The structural changes observed in the brain regions of depressed subjects are shown in the respective boxes.

Source: Sarawagi A, Soni ND and Patel AB (2021) Glutamate and GABA Homeostasis and Neurometabolism in Major Depressive Disorder. Front. Psychiatry 12:637863.

GABA-A receptors, the primary inhibitory receptors in the brain, show altered subunit composition in anxiety and depression. Changes in subunit expression affect receptor pharmacology and function, potentially contributing to reduced inhibitory tone and increased neural excitability in anxiety disorders. These receptor changes may explain individual variation in benzodiazepine response—medications that enhance GABA-A receptor function are more effective when receptors maintain normal subunit composition.

Glutamate receptors undergo extensive modifications in stress-related disorders. NMDA receptors show altered subunit composition, with changes in the ratio of GluN2A to GluN2B subunits affecting receptor kinetics and signaling properties. AMPA receptors, which mediate fast excitatory transmission, show altered expression and reduced synaptic insertion. Metabotropic glutamate receptors, which modulate synaptic function through intracellular signaling cascades, also demonstrate altered expression and function. These glutamate receptor changes contribute to both impaired synaptic plasticity and potential excitotoxicity.

Neuronal Loss and Atrophy

While dendritic changes are reversible and synaptic alterations potentially restorable, severe or prolonged stress and depression can cause irreversible neuronal loss in some brain regions. This represents the most severe form of cellular pathology and contributes to the treatment resistance and chronicity observed in some patients.

Hippocampal volume loss: Magnetic resonance imaging studies consistently demonstrate hippocampal volume reductions in major depression, typically in the range of 8-10% compared to never-depressed individuals. Meta-analyses including thousands of participants confirm this finding across diverse populations and study designs. The volume loss is bilateral but sometimes asymmetric, more pronounced with longer illness duration and more depressive episodes, and partially reversible with successful intervention.

This volume reduction reflects multiple cellular changes. Dendritic atrophy contributes significantly—if dendrites account for substantial neuronal volume, their retraction reduces overall tissue volume without requiring cell death. Reduced neurogenesis in the dentate gyrus means fewer new neurons are added to replace those that naturally die, causing a gradual decline in cell numbers. Reduced glial cell density also contributes to volume loss. However, some degree of actual neuronal death likely occurs, particularly in severe chronic depression.

CA3 pyramidal neurons appear particularly vulnerable to stress-induced death. These neurons possess extensive recurrent connections, making them metabolically demanding and potentially vulnerable to excitotoxicity. Post-mortem studies report reduced CA3 pyramidal cell number in depression, though findings are inconsistent across studies. The extent of frank neuronal death versus severe atrophy without death remains debated, but likely both occur to varying degrees in different individuals.

The functional consequences of hippocampal volume loss are substantial. Memory impairments in depression correlate with hippocampal volume, with smaller hippocampi associated with worse memory performance. The hippocampus's role in regulating HPA axis function becomes compromised, contributing to sustained hypercortisolemia that further damages the hippocampus—a vicious cycle. Impaired pattern separation due to dentate gyrus dysfunction contributes to overgeneralized memory and difficulty distinguishing current situations from past negative experiences.

Critically, hippocampal volume loss is not inevitable or entirely irreversible. Successful intervention can partially restore hippocampal volume, with antidepressant medication, psychotherapy, and exercise all demonstrating volume-increasing effects in some studies. This suggests that significant portions of volume loss reflect functional changes (dendritic atrophy, reduced neurogenesis) rather than irreversible cell death, and that promoting neuroplasticity can restore structure and function.

Prefrontal cortex volume reductions: The prefrontal cortex similarly shows volume reductions in depression, though typically smaller in magnitude than the hippocampus (3-7% reductions). These volume changes are most prominent in the dorsolateral prefrontal cortex, ventromedial prefrontal cortex, and orbitofrontal cortex—regions showing functional hypoactivity in depression.

The cellular basis of prefrontal volume loss includes dendritic atrophy, reduced neuropil (the dense meshwork of dendrites, axons, and glial processes between neuronal cell bodies), decreased glial density, and potentially some degree of neuronal loss. Post-mortem studies reveal reduced neuronal size without consistent evidence of cell number reduction, suggesting that atrophy rather than death predominates. However, glial cells (astrocytes and oligodendrocytes) show more consistent density reductions, indicating that glial pathology contributes significantly to prefrontal volume loss.

Layer-specific changes occur in the prefrontal cortex, with layers III and V showing particular vulnerability. These layers contain pyramidal neurons projecting to other cortical regions and to subcortical structures, respectively. Their dysfunction impairs long-range communication between the prefrontal cortex and other brain regions, potentially explaining the widespread circuit dysfunction observed in depression.

The relationship between prefrontal volume and symptoms is complex. Volume reductions correlate with executive dysfunction, working memory impairment, and psychomotor slowing. However, some symptoms may relate more to functional alterations than structural damage. The dorsolateral prefrontal cortex volume correlates particularly strongly with cognitive symptoms, while ventromedial prefrontal cortex changes relate more to emotional regulation difficulties.

Subgenual anterior cingulate cortex changes: Area 25, the subgenual anterior cingulate cortex, shows particularly prominent alterations in depression. Unlike most regions showing volume reductions, area 25 demonstrates both structural changes and metabolic hyperactivity. The structure shows reduced volume (approximately 30-40% reduction in some studies), reduced glial density (particularly oligodendrocytes and astrocytes), and neuronal atrophy.

The glial loss in area 25 is particularly striking, with some studies reporting 20-40% reductions in glial cell numbers. Since glia outnumber neurons and provide critical support functions, glial loss profoundly affects neural circuit function. Oligodendrocytes that produce myelin are reduced, potentially impairing white matter connections. Astrocytes, which regulate neurotransmitter levels, provide metabolic support, and modulate synaptic function, exhibit both reduced numbers and altered morphology.

The combination of structural volume loss and functional hyperactivity in area 25 seems paradoxical but may reflect a circuit-level compensation—remaining neurons fire excessively, attempting to compensate for overall circuit dysfunction.

This hyperactivity appears maladaptive rather than compensatory, as it correlates with symptom severity and normalizes with successful intervention.

Area 25's role as a critical node coordinating emotional, cognitive, autonomic, and neuroendocrine aspects of depression makes its cellular pathology particularly consequential. Its dysfunction radiates throughout interconnected networks, potentially explaining how localized cellular changes produce such widespread symptomatology.

Other regions: The nucleus accumbens, critical for reward processing and motivation, shows structural changes in depression, including volume reductions and altered cellular morphology. Medium spiny neurons, the principal neurons of the striatum, demonstrate reduced dendritic complexity and spine density in animal depression models. These structural changes provide a cellular substrate for anhedonia and reduced motivation. The amygdala's volume changes in depression and anxiety are complex, with some studies showing increases (possibly reflecting the dendritic hypertrophy discussed previously) and others showing decreases, particularly in chronic conditions. The temporal dynamics may involve initial hypertrophy followed by eventual atrophy as cellular damage accumulates. The thalamus shows volume reductions in some depression studies, potentially reflecting reduced connectivity with cortical regions. The cerebellum, increasingly recognized as relevant to emotional processing beyond motor functions, consistently shows volume alterations in depression, though the functional significance remains unclear.

Neurogenesis Suppression

Adult Neurogenesis Overview

Unlike most brain regions where neurons are generated exclusively during development, the hippocampal dentate gyrus continues producing new neurons throughout life—a process termed adult neurogenesis. Neural stem cells in the subgranular zone of the dentate gyrus divide, producing neuronal precursors that migrate into the granule cell layer, differentiate into mature granule neurons, and integrate into existing circuits. Approximately 700 new neurons are added daily to each human hippocampus, with substantial individual variation.

These adult-born neurons are not merely replacement cells but contribute uniquely to hippocampal function. Young neurons (4-6 weeks post-mitosis) demonstrate heightened excitability and enhanced plasticity compared to mature neurons, making them particularly responsive to learning experiences. They contribute disproportionately to pattern separation—the ability to distinguish between similar experiences or contexts—and to behavioral flexibility. As neurons mature (beyond 8-12 weeks), their properties converge with those of developmentally born neurons. Adult neurogenesis is exquisitely sensitive to environmental and physiological factors. Exercise robustly increases neurogenesis, potentially doubling the production rate. Environmental enrichment—exposure to complex, stimulating environments—enhances neurogenesis and newborn neuron survival. Learning, particularly spatial learning, increases neurogenesis. Social interaction and sexual behavior promote neurogenesis.

Conversely, stress, aging, sleep deprivation, alcohol, and numerous other factors suppress neurogenesis. Chronic stress represents the most potent negative regulator, reducing neurogenesis by 50-80% in animal models. This sensitivity suggests that neurogenesis functions as a plasticity mechanism allowing the hippocampus to adapt to changing environmental demands—increasing capacity during enriched conditions and conserving resources during adversity.

Stress-Induced Neurogenesis Suppression

Chronic stress profoundly suppresses every stage of adult neurogenesis: stem cell proliferation decreases, newly-born cells die at elevated rates, and surviving neurons show impaired differentiation and delayed maturation. The net result is dramatically fewer new neurons integrating into hippocampal circuits.

The mechanisms mediating stress-induced neurogenesis suppression are multifactorial. Glucocorticoids directly suppress neural stem cell proliferation through glucocorticoid receptors expressed by stem cells. Glucocorticoid exposure in vitro reduces stem cell division rates, demonstrating direct cellular effects independent of circuit-level changes. The dentate gyrus's high glucocorticoid receptor density makes it particularly vulnerable to this suppressive effect. Reduced BDNF contributes critically to neurogenesis suppression. BDNF promotes stem cell proliferation, enhances newborn neuron survival, and facilitates dendritic development of maturing neurons. Stress-induced BDNF reduction removes essential neurotrophic support throughout the neurogenic process. Exogenous BDNF administration can partially rescue stress-induced neurogenesis deficits in animal models, demonstrating BDNF's causal role.

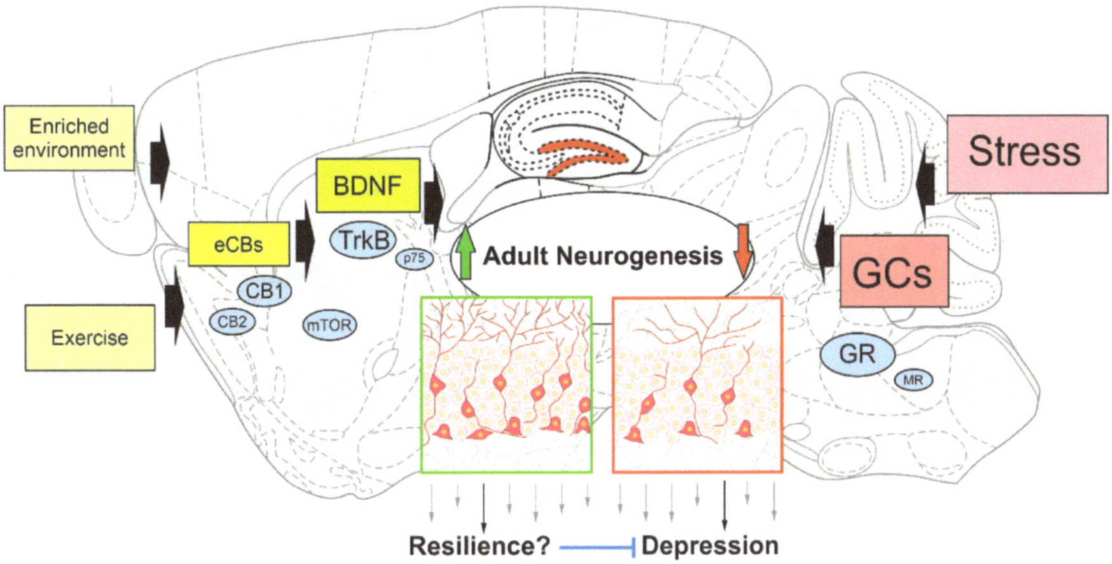

Schematic view of modulating factors of adult hippocampal neurogenesis. Enriched environment, exercise, and molecular players (e.g., endocannabinoids (eCBs) and brain-derived neurotrophic factor (BDNF)) have the potential to upregulate the generation of adult-born neurons in the dentate gyrus. This could confer resilience to the development of depressive-like symptoms through the stress-related decline of adult neurogenesis induced by glucocorticoids (GCs). The main signaling pathways of positive modulators and stress are depicted: cannabinoid receptor type-1 and -2 (CB1; CB2); mammalian target of rapamycin (mTOR); tropomyosin receptor kinase B (TrkB); p75 neurotrophin receptor (p75); glucocorticoid receptor (GR); mineralocorticoid receptor (MR).

Source: Leschik J, Lutz B, Gentile A. Stress-Related Dysfunction of Adult Hippocampal Neurogenesis–An Attempt for Understanding Resilience? International Journal of Molecular Sciences. 2021; 22(14):7339.

Inflammatory processes powerfully suppress neurogenesis. Chronic stress activates hippocampal microglia, which release cytokines including IL-1β, IL-6, and TNF-α. These cytokines directly inhibit neural stem cell proliferation and increase apoptosis of newly-born neurons. Anti-inflammatory interventions prevent stress-induced neurogenesis suppression, and simply administering pro-inflammatory cytokines suppresses neurogenesis even without stress exposure, demonstrating inflammation's sufficient and necessary role.

The inflammatory suppression of neurogenesis may represent an adaptive response in evolutionary contexts—during infection or injury (situations activating immune responses), investing resources in generating new neurons might be maladaptive, and suppressing neurogenesis conserves energy for immune function. However, in chronic psychosocial stress without physical threat, this inflammatory suppression becomes maladaptive, depriving the hippocampus of a critical plasticity mechanism.

Glutamate excitotoxicity affects neurogenesis, with excessive glutamatergic activity in the dentate gyrus increasing cell death among newly-born neurons. The immature neurons lack fully developed mechanisms for buffering calcium influx through NMDA receptors, rendering them particularly vulnerable to excitotoxic death.

Neurotransmitter systems modulate neurogenesis. Serotonin generally promotes proliferation and survival, with serotonin depletion reducing neurogenesis. This may contribute to stress-induced suppression, as stress reduces hippocampal serotonin. Norepinephrine similarly supports neurogenesis, with the locus coeruleus's noradrenergic projections to the hippocampus promoting progenitor proliferation. Dopamine's effects on neurogenesis are complex and context-dependent. GABA provides tonic inhibition, regulating the excitability of the neural stem cell niche.

Vascular factors influence neurogenesis, as neural stem cells reside in close apposition to blood vessels, and the neurovascular niche provides essential signals supporting neurogenesis. Chronic stress reduces hippocampal angiogenesis (new blood vessel formation) and disrupts the neurovascular niche, indirectly compromising neurogenesis. Reduced vascular endothelial growth factor (VEGF) contributes to both impaired angiogenesis and reduced neurogenesis.

The functional consequences of suppressed neurogenesis are debated but appear significant. Animal studies demonstrate that blocking neurogenesis through various means produces depression-like and anxiety-like behaviors. Conversely, increasing neurogenesis through exercise, environmental enrichment, or genetic manipulations produces antidepressant-like and anxiolytic effects. Critically, preventing neurogenesis blocks the behavioral effects of antidepressant medications in some (though not all) animal studies, suggesting that neurogenesis may be necessary for antidepressant efficacy.

Human evidence for neurogenesis's role in depression is necessarily indirect, as directly measuring human hippocampal neurogenesis requires invasive brain tissue sampling. However, post-mortem studies of depressed individuals reveal markers suggesting reduced neurogenesis: fewer neural progenitor cells in the dentate gyrus, reduced expression of proteins associated with immature neurons (doublecortin), and smaller granule cell layer volume (where adult-born neurons reside).

Neurogenesis in Depression and Anxiety

In major depression, the neurogenic hypothesis proposes that impaired hippocampal neurogenesis contributes causally to depressive symptomatology and that antidepressant interventions work partly by restoring neurogenesis. This hypothesis is supported by several lines of evidence:

- **Correlation**: Conditions suppressing neurogenesis (chronic stress, aging, sleep deprivation) increase depression risk, while conditions enhancing neurogenesis (exercise, environmental enrichment, learning) protect against depression.
- **Necessity**: Blocking neurogenesis in animals prevents antidepressant drug effects in some behavioral tests, suggesting neurogenesis is necessary for antidepressant action.
- **Sufficiency**: Enhancing neurogenesis through genetic, viral, or pharmacological approaches produces antidepressant-like effects in animal

models, suggesting neurogenesis is sufficient to improve mood-related behaviors.

- **Time course**: Antidepressant medications typically require 2-4 weeks to produce clinical benefits in humans. This delay matches the time required for newly-born neurons to mature and integrate into circuits in animals, suggesting that neurogenesis's slow time course might explain antidepressants' delayed effects.
- **Treatment response**: Post-mortem studies suggest that antidepressant-treated individuals show markers of enhanced neurogenesis compared to untreated depressed individuals, though interpreting these studies is complicated by multiple confounds. However, the neurogenic hypothesis remains incomplete and controversial. Some antidepressant effects occur too rapidly to involve neurogenesis (ketamine produces antidepressant effects within hours). Not all studies find that blocking neurogenesis prevents antidepressant effects. Human hippocampal neurogenesis rates are significantly lower than those in rodents, raising questions about their clinical relevance. Alternative hypotheses suggest that neurogenesis might mediate some antidepressant effects (particularly on cognitive symptoms and pattern separation) while other mechanisms account for other effects (mood improvement, reduced anhedonia).

In anxiety disorders, reduced neurogenesis appears to contribute to impaired fear extinction and overgeneralized anxiety. Dentate gyrus neurogenesis is critical for pattern separation—distinguishing between similar but distinct contexts. Impaired pattern separation due to reduced neurogenesis could cause overgeneralization of fear—responding anxiously to situations that merely resemble the original threat context rather than representing actual danger.

Animal studies demonstrate that enhancing neurogenesis improves extinction of conditioned fear, while suppressing neurogenesis impairs extinction. This suggests that new neurons may be particularly important for learning that previously feared situations are now safe—a process central to exposure-based anxiety interventions. The overlap between neurogenesis promotion and extinction enhancement suggests potential synergistic approaches combining neurogenesis-enhancing strategies (exercise, environmental enrichment) with extinction-based psychotherapy.

Post-traumatic stress disorder may particularly involve neurogenesis dysfunction. PTSD patients show reduced hippocampal volumes, and combat veterans with PTSD demonstrate markers suggesting impaired neurogenesis. The extinction deficits characteristic of PTSD—difficulty learning that trauma reminders no longer predict danger—could partly reflect inadequate neurogenesis limiting the hippocampus's capacity for new learning.

Glial Cell Alterations

While neuronal dysfunction has dominated psychiatric neuroscience, growing evidence demonstrates that glial cells—astrocytes, oligodendrocytes, and microglia—undergo profound alterations in stress, anxiety, and depression. Given that glia outnumber neurons and perform critical functions supporting neural circuit operation, glial pathology significantly contributes to psychiatric disorders.

Astrocyte Dysfunction

Astrocytes, the most abundant brain cells, perform diverse functions: regulating extracellular neurotransmitter levels through uptake, providing metabolic support to neurons, maintaining the blood-brain barrier, modulating synaptic transmission, and releasing gliotransmitters that influence neuronal activity. Astrocytic dysfunction thus has wide-ranging consequences for circuit function.

Astrocyte density reductions: Post-mortem studies consistently reveal reduced astrocyte density in the prefrontal cortex and hippocampus of individuals with major depression. These reductions range from 10% to 30% depending on the specific region examined and the severity of illness. The orbitofrontal cortex, anterior cingulate cortex, and dorsolateral prefrontal cortex show particularly prominent astrocyte loss.

Reduced astrocyte density does not necessarily indicate cell death—astrocytes may shrink and reduce their territorial domains without dying, making them less detectable in histological studies while still representing true loss of astrocytic function. However, some frank astrocyte death likely occurs with severe chronic stress and depression. The mechanisms include glucocorticoid toxicity, inflammatory cytokine effects, oxidative stress, and withdrawal of neurotrophic support. The functional consequences of reduced astrocyte density are substantial. Each astrocyte contacts thousands of synapses, and astrocyte loss means those synapses lose critical support. Reduced glutamate uptake capacity can lead to excitotoxicity as extracellular glutamate accumulates. Impaired metabolic support compromises neuronal energy supply, particularly during high activity periods. Loss of astrocytic regulation of synaptic transmission alters circuit function.

Morphological alterations: Surviving astrocytes in depression show altered morphology. The extensive processes that astrocytes extend to contact synapses and blood vessels show reduced complexity and branching. This process of retraction reduces the astrocyte's functional territory, specifically the number of synapses and blood vessels it can regulate. Even without cell death, this morphological simplification produces functional astrocyte deficiency. Stress-induced astrocytic atrophy occurs rapidly, within days of chronic stress onset in animal models, preceding neuronal structural changes. This suggests that astrocytic dysfunction may represent an early pathological event that subsequently contributes to neuronal dysfunction. The reversibility of astrocytic morphological changes parallels that of neuronal dendritic changes—with stress removal or antidepressant intervention, astrocytes can re-extend their processes and restore function.

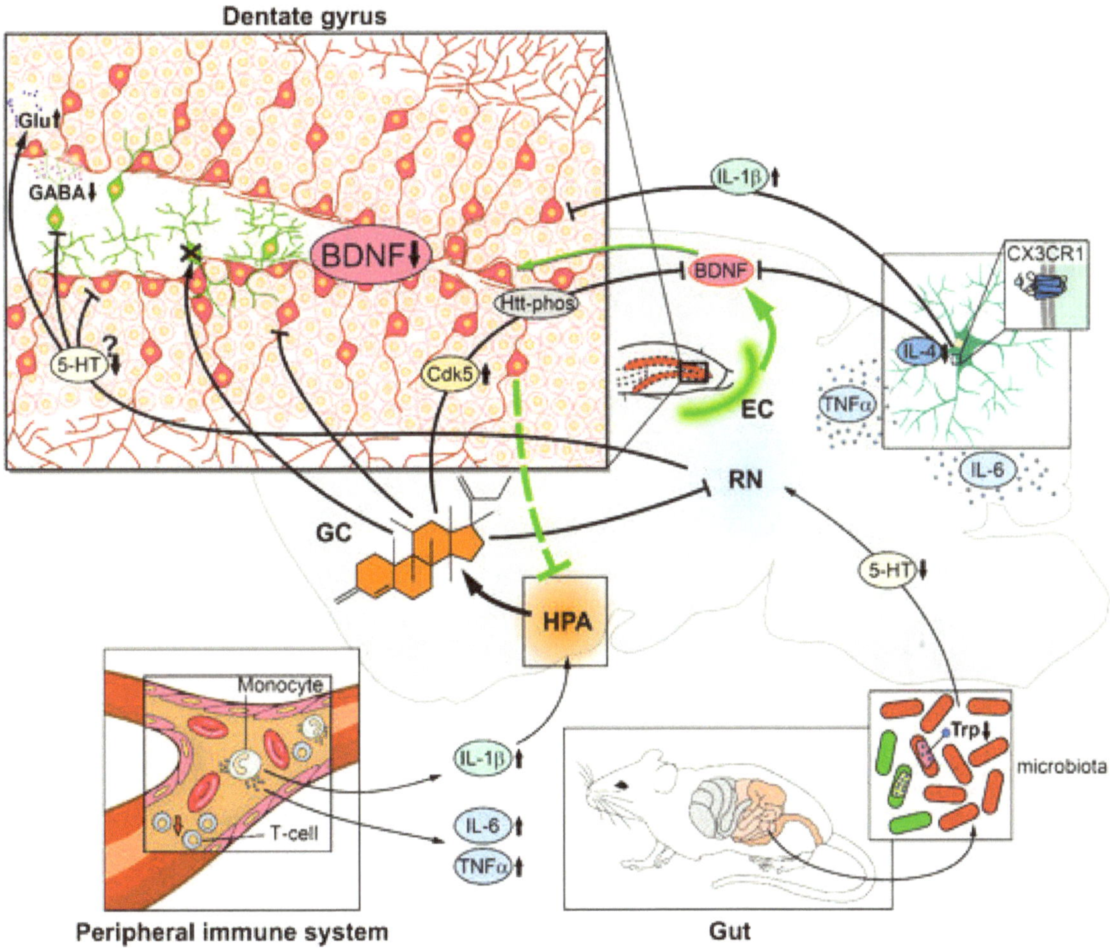

Schematic integrated view of mechanisms conferring negative regulation of adult hippocampal neurogenesis by chronic stress. Hypothalamic-pituitary-adrenal-(HPA) axis controls stress-induced glucocorticoid (GC) release, which exerts a direct negative effect on adult neural stem cells and their progeny (red cells) in the dentate gyrus. In reverse, adult-born neurons exert negative feedback on the HPA axis (green dashed line). HPA axis can get activated by increased interleukin-1β(IL-1β) released by peripheral monocytes. Under conditions of chronic stress, the gut microbiome can change to low tryptophan (Trp) metabolizing microbiota, mainly targeting the serotonergic system of the raphe nuclei (RN), leading to serotonin (5-HT) reduction. 5-HT-reduction might also be due to direct GC effects on raphe neurons, with control of hippocampal glutamatergic and GABAergic release in the dentate gyrus, leading to high glutamate (Glu) and reduced GABA levels. Low GABA is further

caused by a GC-mediated decrease of hilar interneurons (green cells). In addition, reduced 5-HT and dysregulation of 5-HT receptors (5HT1AR and 5HT4R, not depicted) on mature granule cells (light red cells) leading to reduced BDNF availability might be implicated in the stress-induced reduction of neurogenesis. BDNF reduction is also central, due to other mechanisms: (1) Decreased axonal transport of BDNF vesicles from the entorhinal cortex (EC; green arrows for vesicular BDNF-transport), due to hyperphosphorylated huntingtin (Htt-phos) mediated by GC-induced cyclin-dependent kinase 5 (Cdk5); (2) decrease in interleukin-4 (IL-4) sensed by microglia. Moreover, microglia directly inhibit adult neural stem cells and their progeny, (1) through signaling activated by binding of the chemokine CX3CL1 to CX3CR1, which is exclusively expressed on microglia, and (2) by the secretion of IL-1β. Increased interleukin-6 (IL-6) and tumor necrosis factor-α (TNFα) make up the inflammatory milieu of the brain, but are not necessarily released by microglia.

Source: Leschik J, Lutz B, Gentile A. Stress-Related Dysfunction of Adult Hippocampal Neurogenesis–An Attempt for Understanding Resilience? International Journal of Molecular Sciences. 2021; 22(14):7339.

Functional alterations: Beyond structural changes, astrocytes show functional alterations in depression. Glutamate transporter expression, particularly GLT-1 (also called EAAT2), the primary astrocytic glutamate transporter, decreases in depression. Reduced transporter expression impairs glutamate clearance from the synaptic cleft, prolonging glutamate receptor activation and potentially causing excitotoxicity.

The consequences of impaired glutamate uptake extend beyond excitotoxicity. Glutamate spillover from synapses can activate extrasynaptic receptors, which mediate signaling pathways distinct from those of synaptic receptors. This aberrant signaling may contribute to circuit dysfunction. Additionally, glutamate taken up by astrocytes is converted to glutamine and recycled to neurons for neurotransmitter synthesis; impaired uptake thus disrupts the glutamate-glutamine cycle, essential for maintaining neurotransmitter pools.

Astrocytic calcium signaling, through which astrocytes respond to neuronal activity and release gliotransmitters, exhibits alterations in response to stress and depression. This disrupts bidirectional neuron-glia communication, impairing astrocytes' ability to modulate synaptic transmission dynamically. The release of gliotransmitters, including glutamate, ATP, and D-serine, from astrocytes decreases, reducing their participation in synaptic function. Gap junction coupling between astrocytes, which allows them to function as syncytial networks sharing ions and small molecules, becomes disrupted in depression. Connexin proteins forming gap junctions show altered expression. This disconnection of the astrocytic network impairs the spatial buffering of potassium and other ions, thereby reducing the astrocytic network's capacity to maintain an optimal extracellular ionic composition for neuronal function.

Neurotrophic factor production: Astrocytes represent a major source of BDNF and other neurotrophic factors supporting neuronal health. Stress and depression reduce astrocytic BDNF production, contributing to the overall neurotrophic deficit characteristic of these conditions. Since astrocytes contact both neuronal cell bodies and synapses as well as blood vessels, they can integrate diverse signals and deliver neurotrophic support precisely where needed. Loss of this astrocytic neurotrophic function leaves neurons vulnerable to stress-induced damage.

Astrocytes also produce glial cell line-derived neurotrophic factor (GDNF), ciliary neurotrophic factor (CNTF), and other growth factors. The coordinated reduction in multiple neurotrophic factors creates a permissive environment for neuronal dysfunction and degeneration. Interventions that support astrocyte health and function may restore neurotrophic support more effectively than delivering individual growth factors.

Metabolic support dysfunction: Neurons depend on astrocytes for metabolic support, particularly during high activity. The astrocyte-neuron lactate shuttle, in which astrocytes provide lactate to neurons as an energy substrate, becomes impaired in depression. This metabolic coupling dysfunction means neurons have insufficient energy supply during demanding periods, potentially contributing to cognitive dysfunction and fatigue.

Astrocytes also regulate cerebral blood flow through their vascular endfeet, contacting blood vessels. Neurovascular coupling—the process by which local neuronal activity triggers increased blood flow to supply oxygen and glucose—depends on intact astrocytic function. Astrocytic dysfunction disrupts neurovascular coupling, creating mismatches between neuronal energy demand and vascular supply. This may contribute to the vascular abnormalities and altered brain perfusion observed in depression neuroimaging studies.

Oligodendrocyte Alterations

Oligodendrocytes produce myelin, the lipid-rich insulation wrapping axons that enables rapid electrical signal transmission. Beyond simple insulation, oligodendrocytes provide metabolic support to axons, and myelin plasticity contributes to circuit function and learning.

Oligodendrocyte density reductions: Post-mortem studies reveal reduced oligodendrocyte density in the prefrontal cortex, anterior cingulate cortex, and amygdala in depression. These reductions range from 20-40% in some cortical areas, representing a substantial loss of myelinating capacity. The oligodendrocyte loss appears specific rather than reflecting general tissue loss, as neuronal densities often remain normal in regions showing oligodendrocyte depletion.

The mechanisms underlying oligodendrocyte loss include direct glucocorticoid toxicity, as oligodendrocytes express glucocorticoid receptors and chronic glucocorticoid exposure impairs their survival. Inflammatory cytokines, particularly TNF-α and interferon-gamma, are toxic to oligodendrocytes. Oxidative stress and excitotoxicity also damage these cells. Oligodendrocyte precursor cells, which persist throughout adulthood and can differentiate to replace lost oligodendrocytes, show impaired proliferation and differentiation in depression, limiting natural repair mechanisms.

White matter alterations: Diffusion tensor imaging (DTI), an MRI technique assessing white matter microstructure, consistently reveals white matter abnormalities in depression. Fractional anisotropy, a measure of white matter integrity, decreases in multiple white matter tracts, including the anterior limb of the internal capsule, uncinate fasciculus (connecting prefrontal cortex and temporal lobe), cingulum bundle, and corpus callosum.

These white matter changes reflect myelin pathology—reduced myelin thickness, irregular myelin structure, or loss of myelinated axons. Since white matter tracts mediate communication between brain regions, white matter pathology disrupts long-range connectivity. The disrupted fronto-limbic connectivity characteristic of depression—impaired communication between prefrontal regulatory regions and limbic emotional regions—may partly reflect white matter/myelin pathology rather than (or in addition to) gray matter dysfunction.

The relationship between white matter abnormalities and symptoms is emerging. Executive dysfunction correlates with frontal white matter integrity. Processing speed reductions correlate with widespread white matter changes. The severity and extent of white matter abnormalities predict treatment response, with more extensive abnormalities associated with poorer outcomes and treatment resistance.

Myelin plasticity impairment: Beyond maintaining existing myelin, oligodendrocytes demonstrate plasticity—modifying myelin thickness and even myelinating previously unmyelinated axons in response to neuronal activity and learning. This myelin plasticity contributes to circuit optimization and skill acquisition. Stress and depression impair myelin plasticity, potentially contributing to cognitive inflexibility and difficulty learning new adaptive responses.

Activity-dependent myelination, in which increased neuronal activity stimulates increased myelination of those neurons' axons, becomes disrupted in depression. This impairs the brain's capacity to strengthen important connections through experience-dependent myelin modification. The reduced behavioral flexibility and perseverative negative thinking characteristic of depression may partly reflect impaired myelin plasticity, limiting circuit reorganization.

Metabolic consequences: Oligodendrocytes provide metabolic support to axons, delivering lactate and other metabolites that support axonal energy metabolism. The myelin sheath itself serves metabolic functions beyond insulation. Oligodendrocyte loss thus impairs axonal energy metabolism, potentially contributing to axonal dysfunction and degeneration even before demyelination becomes apparent.

The high metabolic demands of maintaining myelin mean that oligodendrocytes are vulnerable to metabolic stress. The reduced cerebral glucose metabolism observed in depression may particularly affect oligodendrocytes, contributing to their dysfunction. This creates a vicious cycle where oligodendrocyte dysfunction impairs circuit function, reducing activity and metabolism, which further compromises oligodendrocyte health.

Microglial Activation

Microglia, the brain's resident immune cells, exist in ramified "resting" states during health, with extensively branched processes surveying the local environment. Upon detecting pathology - infection, injury, cellular debris, or inflammatory signals—microglia become activated, retracting processes, proliferating, and releasing inflammatory mediators. Microglial activation represents a double-edged sword: acute activation supports tissue repair, but chronic activation causes neuroinflammation and neuronal damage.

Chronic microglial activation: Multiple lines of evidence demonstrate microglial activation in depression. Positron emission tomography (PET) imaging using tracers that bind to the translocator protein (TSPO), a marker upregulated in activated microglia, reveals increased signal in the brains of individuals with depression. This increase appears most prominent in the anterior cingulate cortex, prefrontal cortex, and insula, correlating with symptom severity.

Post-mortem studies confirm microglial activation, with morphological analyses revealing that microglia in the brains of individuals with depression exhibit an activated morphology, characterized by reduced process branching, enlarged cell bodies, and increased cell density. Markers of activation, including MHC-II and CD11b, exhibit elevated expression. The pattern suggests chronic low-grade activation rather than acute intense activation—a "primed" or "sensitized" state where microglia overreact to minor stimuli.

The triggers for microglial activation in depression include chronic stress signals, peripheral inflammatory cytokines crossing the blood-brain barrier or signaling through circumventricular organs, damage-associated molecular patterns (DAMPs) released from stressed neurons, and a disrupted blood-brain barrier allowing entry of peripheral immune components. Psychosocial stress activates peripheral immune cells, which release inflammatory mediators that reach the brain and activate microglia.

Pro-inflammatory cytokine production: Activated microglia release pro-inflammatory cytokines, including interleukin-1β (IL-1β), interleukin-6 (IL-6), tumor necrosis factor-alpha (TNF-α), and others. These cytokines have profound effects on neuronal function even without causing frank neurotoxicity.

IL-1β impairs long-term potentiation, disrupting synaptic plasticity and learning. It reduces BDNF expression, contributing to neurotrophic deficiency. IL-1β affects neurotransmitter metabolism, reducing serotonin synthesis while increasing serotonin reuptake, creating a neurochemical profile resembling depression. It activates the HPA axis, contributing to hypercortisolemia.

TNF-α increases glutamate release while impairing glutamate reuptake by astrocytes, creating conditions for excitotoxicity. It reduces synaptic strength by increasing AMPA receptor internalization, weakening excitatory synapses. TNF-α impairs neurogenesis, contributing to suppressed hippocampal plasticity.

IL-6, while having some neuroprotective effects in acute contexts, becomes deleterious when chronically elevated. It affects neurotransmitter metabolism, particularly reducing dopamine synthesis, potentially contributing to anhedonia and fatigue. IL-6 correlates strongly with depression severity in clinical studies.

These cytokines create a neuroinflammatory milieu that impairs neuroplasticity, disrupts neurotransmitter systems, suppresses neurogenesis, and promotes neuronal dysfunction. The inflammatory hypothesis of depression proposes that this cytokine-mediated neuroinflammation represents a core pathological mechanism in at least a substantial subset of depressed individuals.

Neurotoxic effects: Beyond cytokine release, chronically activated microglia produce reactive oxygen species (ROS) and reactive nitrogen species (RNS), including nitric oxide and superoxide. These reactive molecules cause oxidative and nitrosative stress, damaging proteins, lipids, and DNA. Neurons are particularly vulnerable to oxidative damage due to high metabolic rates, abundant oxidizable lipids in membranes, and relatively limited antioxidant defenses.

Chronic microglial activation can progress to a neurotoxic phenotype sometimes termed "M1" activation (though microglial activation states exist on a continuum rather than discrete categories). Neurotoxic microglia produce quinolinic acid, a neurotoxic tryptophan metabolite that activates NMDA receptors and causes excitotoxicity. This shifts tryptophan metabolism away from serotonin synthesis (as tryptophan is diverted to the kynurenine pathway, producing quinolinic acid), simultaneously reducing serotonin production and increasing neurotoxic metabolites.

Activated microglia also phagocytose synapses, a process termed "synaptic pruning" that is adaptive during development but becomes pathological when excessive in adulthood. Chronic stress and inflammation induce excessive microglial synaptic pruning, contributing to synaptic loss in depression. The complement system, part of the innate immune system, tags synapses for microglial elimination, and this system shows altered activity in depression.

Impaired neuroprotective functions: Microglia can also adopt neuroprotective phenotypes (sometimes termed "M2"), releasing anti-inflammatory cytokines (IL-10, TGF-β), producing neurotrophic factors, and supporting tissue repair. In depression, this protective microglial function appears to be impaired - microglia remain stuck in pro-inflammatory states rather than transitioning into reparative phenotypes.

The balance between neurotoxic and neuroprotective microglial states depends on local environmental signals. In healthy conditions, microglia transition flexibly between states as needed. In chronic stress and depression, this flexibility is lost, and microglia remain chronically activated in pro-inflammatory states that perpetuate rather than resolve pathology.

Inflammatory heterogeneity: Not all individuals with depression show evidence of inflammation—approximately 30-40% of depressed individuals show elevated peripheral inflammatory markers, while others have normal or even reduced inflammation. This suggests that depression comprises heterogeneous conditions, with an "inflammatory subtype" driven primarily by immune dysfunction and other subtypes involving different primary mechanisms. The inflammatory subtype of depression shows distinctive features: elevated C-reactive protein (CRP), IL-6, and TNF-α in peripheral blood; greater treatment resistance to conventional antidepressants; possible preferential response to anti-inflammatory approaches; more prominent symptoms of fatigue, anhedonia, and psychomotor slowing; and often comorbidity with medical conditions involving inflammation (obesity, cardiovascular disease, autoimmune conditions). Identifying inflammatory depression through biomarkers could enable personalized approaches targeting inflammation specifically in those who would benefit. Anti-inflammatory medications, immunomodulatory interventions, or even lifestyle modifications addressing inflammation (exercise, diet, stress reduction) might particularly help this subgroup.

Neural Stem Cells and Cellular Approach

The Neural Stem cell (NSC) approach represents a frontier in neuropsychiatric treatment, with potential applications targeting structural damage, neurochemical dysfunction, and inflammatory processes underlying stress, anxiety, and depression.

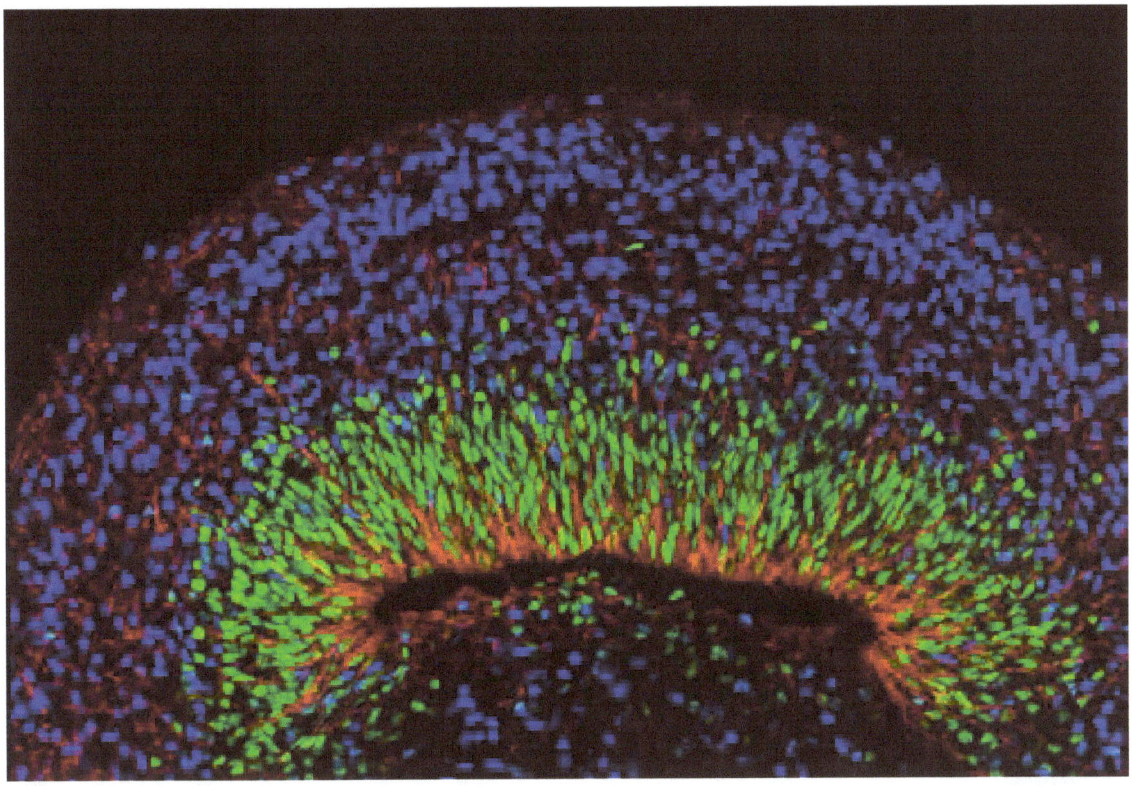

A microscope image of a mini brain organoid showing layered neural tissue and different types of neural cells. | Credit: UCLA Broad Stem Cell Research Center/Nature Neuroscience

The structural and functional brain alterations in stress-related psychiatric disorders—hippocampal atrophy, prefrontal cortex volume loss, reduced neurogenesis, glial dysfunction, and inflammatory activation—suggest that regenerative approaches might address root pathophysiological processes rather than merely ameliorating symptoms. NSC offers theoretical potential to:

- **Replace damaged or lost neurons**: Differentiated NSCs could theoretically replace neurons lost to chronic stress or depression, particularly in the hippocampus and prefrontal cortex, where structural deficits are prominent.
- **Enhance endogenous neurogenesis** NSCs - derived factors could stimulate the brain's intrinsic neurogenic capacity, particularly in the hippocampal dentate gyrus, where adult neurogenesis continues throughout life.
- **Provide neurotrophic support**: NSCs secrete brain-derived neurotrophic factor (BDNF), nerve growth factor (NGF), and other neurotrophins that support neuronal survival, promote dendritic arborization, enhance synaptic plasticity, and facilitate the reorganization of neural circuits.
- **Modulate neuroinflammation**: Certain NSCs types demonstrate immunomodulatory properties, potentially reducing the neuroinflammatory processes implicated in depression and stress-related disorders.
- **Restore glial function**: NSCs could differentiate into astrocytes and oligodendrocytes, addressing the glial deficits documented in depression.

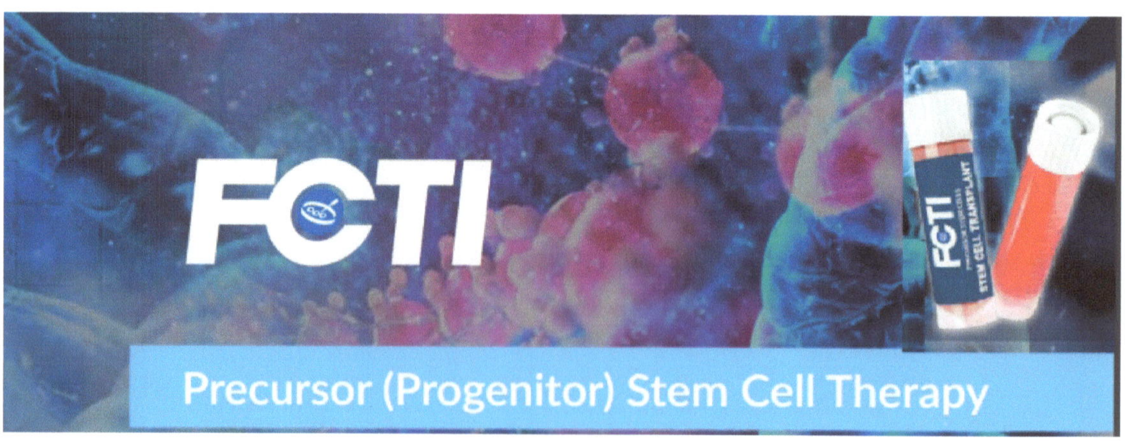

Source: product courtesy FCTI R & D Laboratories GMBH, Germany & Baden Research, Germany

Brain Structures Involved in Stress, Anxiety, and Depression

The neurobiology of stress, anxiety, and depression involves a complex network of interconnected brain structures spanning cortical, subcortical, and brainstem regions. These structures operate as integrated circuits rather than isolated modules, with extensive reciprocal connections enabling coordinated responses to environmental challenges and internal states. Understanding the anatomical substrates and functional roles of these regions provides essential context for comprehending the pathophysiology of stress-related psychiatric conditions and potential therapeutic interventions.

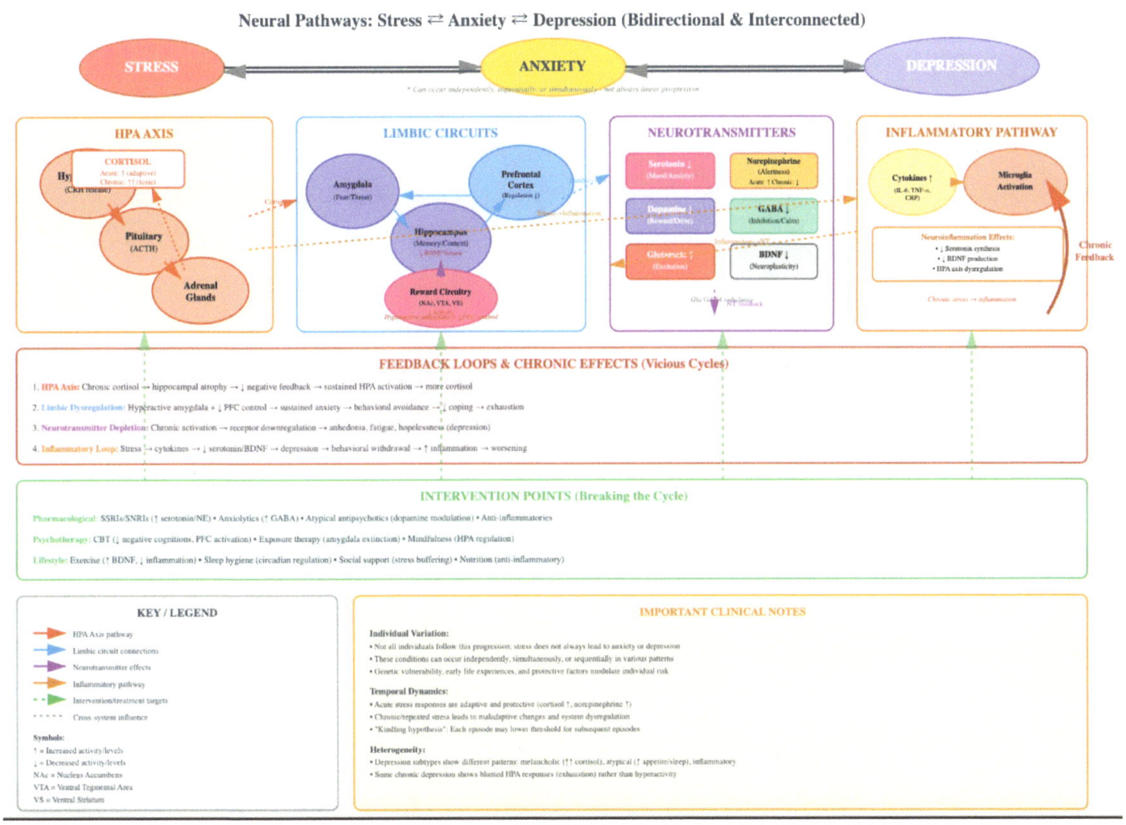

Modern research emphasizes that chronic stress leads to inflammation and then to depression. As such, the cytokine hypothesis (IL-6, TNF-α, CRP affecting brain function) is a major contemporary model.

- *Reward circuitry:* While dopamine is mentioned, the ventral tegmental area (VTA), nucleus accumbens, and ventral striatum—critical for anhedonia in depression - are explicitly shown in the limbic circuits section.
- *Neuroplasticity changes:* BDNF (brain-derived neurotrophic factor) reduction and impaired neurogenesis in the hippocampus are key mechanisms

NSCs Amygdala

The amygdala comprises a collection of nuclei located in the medial temporal lobe, anterior to the hippocampus. This almond-shaped structure (its name derives from the Greek word for almond) consists of approximately 13 distinct nuclei organized into three main functional groups: the basolateral complex (lateral, basal, and accessory basal nuclei), the cortical-like group (cortical nuclei and nucleus of the lateral olfactory tract), and the centromedial group (central and medial nuclei). The basolateral amygdala receives highly processed sensory information from association cortices and the thalamus, enabling integration of complex environmental stimuli. The central nucleus serves as the primary output station, projecting to hypothalamic, brainstem, and autonomic structures that mediate emotional responses. The medial nucleus connects with the olfactory system and plays roles in social and reproductive behaviors.

Amygdala's NSCs may participate in maintaining the cellular adaptability of networks involved in emotional threat detection and fear-learning processes. Because the amygdala responds rapidly to potential danger, the presence of regenerative cells could support the stability of these survival-oriented circuits. Experimental data suggest that NSCs might help sustain the amygdala's ability to manage fast emotional responses to environmental changes.

The NSCs of the amygdala can contribute to emotional salience processing by helping prioritize experiences with strong emotional relevance. This may include both positive and negative events that shape memory and attention. Their influence might allow emotional learning to remain flexible and responsive to new contexts, which is important for adapting to stressors over time.

Advantages in Stress, Anxiety & Depression:

- Sustain rapid threat evaluation while allowing flexible updating of fear responses
- Support fear extinction learning, helping reduce inappropriate or persistent anxiety
- Maintain sensitivity to social and emotional cues, preventing excessive withdrawal or distrust
- Counteract overstimulation of the amygdala that contributes to chronic vigilance and emotional hyperreactivity

This regenerative capability preserves balanced emotional salience and protects against pathological fear conditioning common in anxiety disorders.

Studies indicate that stress hormones can strongly influence amygdala reactivity. NSCs of the amygdala in this region may provide cellular support against potential negative consequences of prolonged stress, such as heightened vigilance or exaggerated fear responses. This potential regenerative element could be significant in anxiety-related behaviors where threat evaluation becomes overly sensitive.

In disorders such as major depression, changes in social signal interpretation are often observed. Amygdala's NSCs might support the preservation of responsiveness to emotionally relevant facial expressions and interpersonal cues. By enabling ongoing circuit refinement, they may help prevent rigid or maladaptive emotional states that contribute to anxiety and depressive symptoms.

NSCs Hippocampus

The hippocampus is a seahorse-shaped structure (its name derives from the Greek for seahorse) located in the medial temporal lobe, posterior to the amygdala. It consists of several subregions: the dentate gyrus (site of ongoing adult neurogenesis), CA3 (providing recurrent connections supporting pattern completion), CA1 (the primary hippocampal output), CA2, and the subiculum. The hippocampus receives highly processed polymodal sensory information via the entorhinal cortex and projects back to cortical regions, forming a critical component of memory systems. It maintains extensive bidirectional connections with the amygdala, enabling emotional modulation of memory and contextual regulation of emotional responses.

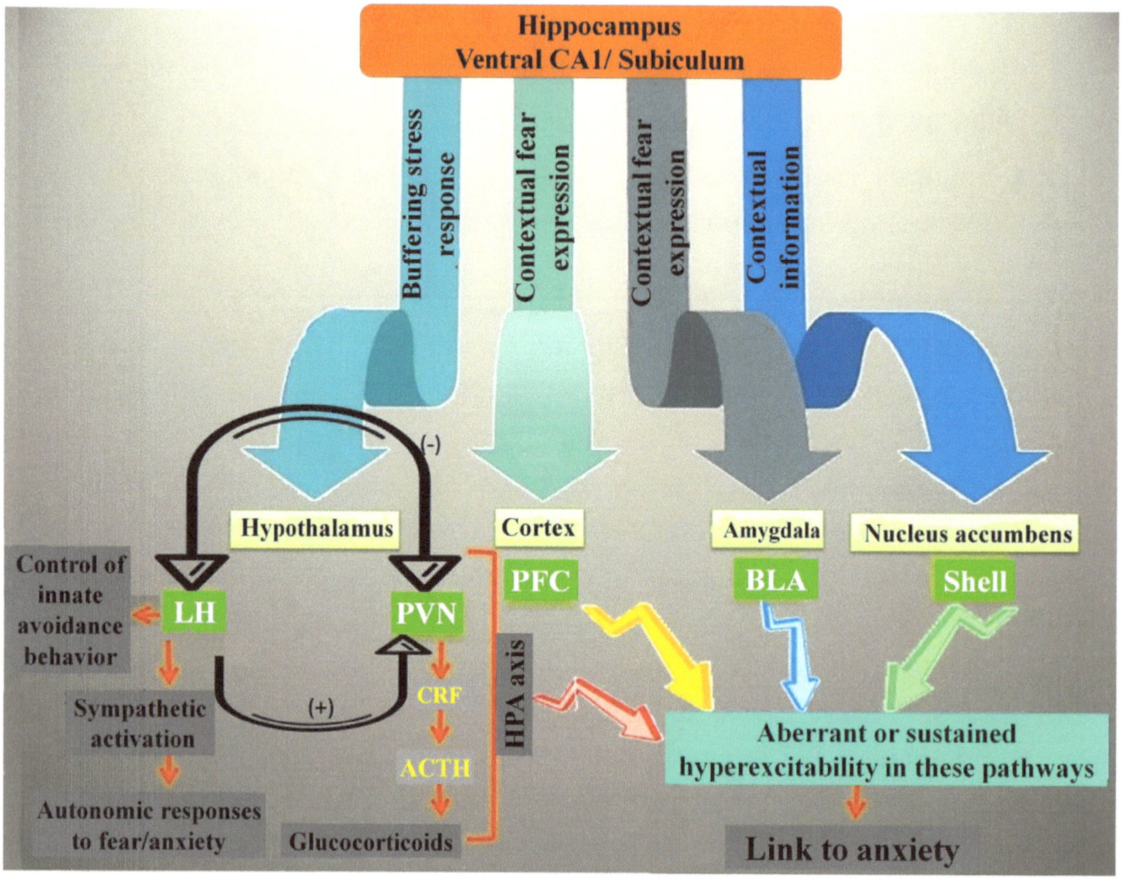

Association between the hippocampal activity and brain regions involved in anxiety. Source: Ghasemi, M., et al. Anxiety and hippocampal neuronal activity: Relationship and potential mechanisms. Cogn Affect Behav Neurosci 22, 431–449 (2022).

The hippocampus serves as the brain's cognitive map, encoding spatial information, temporal sequences, and contextual details of experiences. It is essential for declarative memory formation (explicit memory for facts and events) and consolidates memories from short-term to long-term storage through interactions with cortical regions. In the context of stress and emotion, the hippocampus provides contextual information that modulates emotional responses. It enables discrimination between safe and dangerous contexts, helps determine whether current situations resemble past threatening experiences, and supports extinction learning (learning that previously dangerous situations are now safe). The hippocampus expresses high concentrations of glucocorticoid receptors, making it particularly sensitive to stress hormones. This sensitivity serves adaptive functions in modulating learning during stress but also renders the structure vulnerable to damage from chronic stress exposure. The dentate gyrus undergoes ongoing neurogenesis throughout life, a process that appears important for certain forms of learning, mood regulation, and stress resilience—and is notably suppressed by chronic stress and depression.

The hippocampus represents a particularly compelling target for NSCs interventions given its documented structural deficits in depression and chronic stress, ongoing endogenous neurogenesis throughout life, critical roles in stress regulation, contextual memory, and mood, and relative accessibility for localized interventions. Several studies of NSCs of the hippocampus have demonstrated their integration into existing neural circuits, differentiation of stem cells into functional granule neurons, behavioral improvements, including reduced anxiety-like and depression-like behaviors, enhanced spatial memory and cognitive function, and increased endogenous neurogenesis. These effects appear to be mediated by both direct neuronal replacement and neurotrophic factors secreted by NSCs, which enhance the survival and function of existing neurons. NSCs of the hippocampus increase BDNF levels in the hippocampus, promoting neuroplasticity and potentially reversing stress-induced dendritic atrophy.

The hippocampal NSCs may also support the formation of new neurons involved in memory processing, contextual learning, and the regulation of emotional significance. This is particularly relevant because chronic stress can affect hippocampal structure and function. During stress-related disorders, cortisol exposure has been shown to impair hippocampal volume and memory performance. Hippocampal NSCs may provide a mechanism for structural recovery by supporting the replacement of vulnerable neurons. In this regard, boosting NSC activity could help counteract stress-induced cognitive decline observed in depression.

Research suggests that hippocampal neurogenesis might influence serotonin-regulated pathways associated with mood stabilization. NSCs in this region may contribute to the processes underlying resilience and coping strategies. This could be particularly important in disorders where individuals experience repetitive negative thinking or reduced ability to learn from supportive experiences. Fear generalization—a feature common in anxiety—is often linked to impaired hippocampal function. By supporting accurate contextual memory, hippocampal NSCs might help the brain distinguish harmless environments from true threats. This potential for improved discrimination may reduce excessive or prolonged anxiety responses.

Mechanisms of action: NSCs of the hippocampus could:

- Restore granule neuron populations in the dentate gyrus depleted by chronic stress
- Enhance pattern separation capacity, improving contextual discrimination
- Strengthen negative feedback on the HPA axis, normalizing stress hormone regulation
- Improve hippocampal-prefrontal connectivity, enhancing emotion regulation
- Increase BDNF and other neurotrophins, promoting widespread neural plasticity
- In stress, hippocampal NSCs may help restore the hippocampal volume reduced by high cortisol levels
- In anxiety, NSCs might improve discrimination between safe and threatening cues, reducing generalized fear
- In depression, they can support mood-regulating pathways involving serotonin and neurotrophic factors such as BDNF

Their contribution to neuroplasticity could represent a protective mechanism against cognitive decline and hopelessness associated with mood disorders.

Major Brain Structures and Their Involvement

Brain Structure	Location/ Anatomy	Role in Stress	Role in Anxiety	Role in Depression	Structural Changes	Functional Changes	Management Targets	Stem Cell Potential
Hippocampus	Medial temporal lobe; includes dentate gyrus, CA1-CA3, subiculum	Contextual evaluation of stressors; negative feedback on HPA axis; memory consolidation for stressful events	Contextual processing of threats; pattern separation between safe/dangerous contexts; extinction learning	Impaired contextual memory; reduced negative feedback on HPA axis; overgeneralized autobiographical memory	Volume reduction (8-10%); dendritic atrophy; reduced neurogenesis in dentate gyrus; CA3 pyramidal cell loss	Reduced activation during memory encoding; impaired extinction recall; weakened connectivity with PFC and amygdala	SSRIs increase neurogenesis; cognitive therapy enhances extinction; exercise promotes BDNF	Adult neurogenesis site; accessible for NSC transplantation; proven preclinical efficacy; dentate gyrus restoration

Brain Structure	Location/ Anatomy	Role in Stress	Role in Anxiety	Role in Depression	Structural Changes	Functional Changes	Management Targets	Stem Cell Potential
Amygdala	Medial temporal lobe; basolateral complex, central nucleus, medial nucleus	Rapid threat detection; emotional salience assignment; initiates HPA axis and autonomic responses	Hyperactive fear processing; excessive threat detection; heightened response to ambiguous stimuli	Negative emotional bias; enhanced responses to negative stimuli; reduced responses to positive stimuli	Increased volume in anxiety; variable in depression; dendritic growth with chronic stress	Hyperreactivity to threats; impaired habituation; increased connectivity with insula and subgenual ACC	Exposure therapy promotes extinction; SSRIs reduce reactivity; propranolol blocks reconsolidation	Hyperactivity rather than loss; potential GABAergic interneuron enhancement; modulating rather than replacing
Prefrontal Cortex (General)	Anterior frontal lobes; ~30% of cortex	Cognitive appraisal of stressors; top-down emotion regulation; stress coping strategies	Regulatory control over amygdala; cognitive reappraisal; inhibition of worry and avoidance	Executive dysfunction; impaired emotion regulation; reduced cognitive control; rumination	Reduced gray matter volume; cortical thinning; decreased dendritic complexity; synaptic loss	Hypoactivation during cognitive tasks; reduced connectivity with limbic regions; impaired working memory	Cognitive therapy strengthens prefrontal function; TMS enhances activity; stimulants improve cognition	Complex connectivity requirements; multiple subtypes needed; glial support may be more feasible

Brain Structure	Location/ Anatomy	Role in Stress	Role in Anxiety	Role in Depression	Structural Changes	Functional Changes	Management Targets	Stem Cell Potential
Dorsolateral PFC (dlPFC)	Lateral surface of frontal lobes (areas 9, 46)	Working memory maintenance during stress; cognitive flexibility; planning under pressure	Cognitive control over attention to threat; reappraisal of anxiety-provoking situations	Impaired working memory; reduced concentration; difficulty with planning and decision-making	Reduced volume; cortical thinning particularly in left hemisphere	Hypoactivation during executive tasks; reduced connectivity with parietal cortex	TMS targeting (FDA-approved for depression); cognitive remediation; stimulant medications	Long-range connectivity critical; layer-specific pyramidal neurons needed; trophic support more realistic
Ventromedial PFC (vmPFC)	Medial and orbital frontal surfaces (areas 10, 11, 14, 25, 32)	Integration of emotional and cognitive information; value-based decision-making under stress	Fear extinction consolidation; safety signal processing; inhibition of amygdala	Negative self-referential processing; impaired reward valuation; autonomic dysregulation	Reduced volume in subgenual region; altered connectivity	Reduced activation during extinction recall; increased connectivity with amygdala in depression	Extinction-based therapies; mindfulness strengthens vmPFC; area 25 DBS for treatment-resistant depression	Extinction circuit target; potential for enhancing inhibitory control; immunomodulation of area 25

Brain Structure	Location/ Anatomy	Role in Stress	Role in Anxiety	Role in Depression	Structural Changes	Functional Changes	Management Targets	Stem Cell Potential
Anterior Cingulate Cortex (ACC)	Medial frontal lobe surrounding corpus callosum (areas 24, 32, 33)	Conflict monitoring; error detection; pain processing during stress	Excessive performance monitoring; hypervigilance for errors and threats	Rumination maintenance (subgenual); autonomic dysregulation; reduced motivation	Reduced subgenual ACC volume in familial depression	Dorsal ACC hyperactivity in anxiety; subgenual hyperactivity in depression correlates with rumination	Area 25 (subgenual) DBS; mindfulness reduces ACC hyperactivity; SSRIs normalize metabolism	Subgenual ACC (area 25) specific target; immunomodulation may reduce hyperactivity; connectivity modulation
Orbitofrontal Cortex (OFC)	Inferior frontal surface above orbits (areas 11, 13, 14, 47)	Reward/ punishment evaluation; adaptive behavior adjustment based on outcomes	Altered threat-reward trade-offs; excessive avoidance despite potential rewards	Reduced reward sensitivity; impaired value representation; maladaptive decision-making	Volume reductions in lateral OFC	Altered responses to rewards and punishments; impaired reversal learning	Cognitive therapy addressing cognitive distortions; reward-focused interventions	Complex reward circuitry; multiple target regions; trophic support more feasible than replacement

Brain Structure	Location/ Anatomy	Role in Stress	Role in Anxiety	Role in Depression	Structural Changes	Functional Changes	Management Targets	Stem Cell Potential
Nucleus Accumbens (NAc)	Ventral striatum at caudate-putamen junction; core and shell subdivisions	Stress affects reward processing; motivation for coping behaviors; stress-induced anhedonia	Variable—can show normal reward responses unlike in depression	Profound anhedonia; reduced motivation; blunted responses to rewards; reduced anticipatory pleasure	Reduced volume with chronic stress/ depression; altered dendritic spine density	Hypoactivation to rewards; reduced dopamine release; impaired reward learning	Behavioral activation therapy; potentially dopamine agonists; ketamine restores reward responses	Critical for anhedonia; MSC-derived factors might enhance dopamine; behavioral interventions synergistic
Ventral Tegmental Area (VTA)	Midbrain; source of mesolimbic and mesocortical dopamine projections	Stress affects dopamine signaling; chronic stress reduces tonic dopamine	Typically preserved dopamine function	Reduced dopamine neuron firing; decreased dopamine synthesis and release	Possible neuronal loss with severe chronic stress	Reduced tonic and phasic dopamine signaling; blunted responses to rewards	Dopamine agonists (limited efficacy); behavioral activation; exercise increases dopamine	Dopamine neuron replacement theoretically beneficial; neurotrophic support; challenges in axon guidance to targets

Brain Structure	Location/ Anatomy	Role in Stress	Role in Anxiety	Role in Depression	Structural Changes	Functional Changes	Management Targets	Stem Cell Potential
Hypothalamus	Base of brain forming floor of third ventricle; multiple nuclei including PVN, SCN, arcuate	CENTRAL: PVN releases CRH initiating HPA axis; coordinates neuroendocrine and autonomic responses	Sustained HPA activation via BNST inputs; autonomic hyperarousal	HPA axis hyperactivity; CRH overproduction; impaired negative feedback; circadian rhythm disruption	CRH neuron hypertrophy; altered receptor expression	PVN hyperactivity; reduced glucocorticoid receptor sensitivity; SCN circadian dysfunction	CRH receptor antagonists (experimental); cortisol synthesis inhibitors; circadian interventions	Small, complex nuclei; critical functions risk disruption; modulation safer than replacement
Pituitary Gland	Sella turcica below hypothalamus; anterior and posterior divisions	ACTH release in response to CRH; amplification of stress signal	Sustained ACTH elevation with chronic anxiety	Hypercortisolemia via excessive ACTH; impaired dexamethasone suppression	Corticotroph hyperplasia with chronic stress	Increased ACTH secretion; reduced sensitivity to negative feedback	Targeting upstream (CRH) or downstream (cortisol synthesis) more common than pituitary itself	Endocrine organ; systemic effects; replacement impractical and unnecessary

Brain Structure	Location/ Anatomy	Role in Stress	Role in Anxiety	Role in Depression	Structural Changes	Functional Changes	Management Targets	Stem Cell Potential
Adrenal Glands	Above kidneys; cortex produces cortisol	Cortisol synthesis and release; mobilizes energy; modulates immune function	Sustained cortisol elevation in chronic anxiety states	Hypercortisolemia (most patients) or hypocortisolemia (some with chronic depression—exhaustion)	Adrenal hypertrophy with chronic stress	Increased cortisol production; altered circadian rhythm; variable sensitivity to ACTH	Cortisol synthesis inhibitors (mifepristone for psychotic depression); mineralocorticoid receptor antagonists	Peripheral endocrine organ; not brain structure; not target for neuropsychiatric stem cells
Thalamus	Central brain; relay station surrounding third ventricle; multiple nuclei	Sensory relay including threat-related information; arousal modulation	Heightened sensory processing; threat information relay to amygdala and cortex	Disrupted connectivity with PFC and limbic regions; altered sensory processing	Volume reductions reported in some studies	Altered connectivity patterns; disrupted thalamo-cortical rhythms	Indirect via improving cortical function; thalamic TMS experimental	Relay station; multiple nuclei with distinct functions; connectivity target rather than replacement

Brain Structure	Location/ Anatomy	Role in Stress	Role in Anxiety	Role in Depression	Structural Changes	Functional Changes	Management Targets	Stem Cell Potential
Insula	Buried in lateral sulcus beneath opercula; posterior to anterior gradient	Interoceptive awareness; physiological arousal detection; pain processing	HIGH: Interoceptive amplification; heightened awareness of autonomic arousal; disgust processing	Somatic symptoms; altered interoceptive processing; increased sensitivity to pain and discomfort	Variable structural findings	Hyperactivation in anxiety (especially panic); altered activation patterns in depression	Interoceptive exposure therapy; mindfulness reduces insula hyperactivity	Complex integration hub; connectivity-based dysfunction; modulation more relevant than replacement
Bed Nucleus of Stria Terminalis (BNST)	Basal forebrain; part of extended amygdala	Sustained anxiety responses; uncertainty processing	CRITICAL: Sustained anxiety to unpredictable/ distant threats; hypervigilance maintenance	Contributes to sustained negative affect; anxiety component of depression	Altered connectivity with amygdala and hypothalamus	Hyperactivity in anxiety disorders; sustained CRH release; enhanced threat vigilance	Anxiolytics may reduce BNST activation; CRH receptor antagonists; no specific approved approaches	Small structure; extended amygdala; connectivity-based; modulation preferable to cell replacement

Brain Structure	Location/ Anatomy	Role in Stress	Role in Anxiety	Role in Depression	Structural Changes	Functional Changes	Management Targets	Stem Cell Potential
Periaqueductal Gray (PAG)	Midbrain surrounding cerebral aqueduct; dorsal, lateral, ventrolateral columns	Defensive behavior coordination; pain modulation; freeze/ flight/fight responses	PANIC: Hyperactivity triggers panic attacks; suffocation alarm sensitivity	Altered pain processing; freeze responses; potential role in psychomotor changes	Minimal structural changes documented	Hyperactivity in panic disorder; altered defensive behavior organization	Panic disorder medications (SSRIs, benzodiazepines) likely affect PAG; no direct targeting	Brainstem; critical defensive functions; intervention risks severe dysfunction
Locus Coeruleus (LC)	Dorsal pons; small bilateral nuclei	MAJOR: Norepinephrine release; arousal; vigilance; facilitates memory for stressful events	Hyperactivity contributes to hypervigilance and autonomic symptoms	Variable: hyperactivity in anxious depression; hypoactivity in psychomotor retardation	Possible volume loss in severe depression	Altered firing patterns; dysregulated norepinephrine release; abnormal circadian activity	SNRIs increase norepinephrine; alpha-2 agonists reduce LC firing; atomoxetine in comorbid ADHD	Brainstem; widespread projections; small nuclei; noradrenergic identity critical; replacement impractical

Brain Structure	Location/ Anatomy	Role in Stress	Role in Anxiety	Role in Depression	Structural Changes	Functional Changes	Management Targets	Stem Cell Potential
Raphe Nuclei	Brainstem midline from midbrain to medulla; dorsal and median raphe primary	Serotonin release modulates stress responses; stress affects serotonergic function	Reduced serotonergic tone contributes to anxiety; 5-HT1A receptor dysfunction	CRITICAL: Serotonergic dysfunction central to depression; reduced 5-HT synthesis and release	Reduced raphe volume; neuronal loss in suicide victims	Reduced serotonin neuron firing; altered receptor expression; impaired synthesis	SSRIs primary target; 5-HT1A agonists; tryptophan supplementation	Brainstem; serotonergic identity maintenance challenging; extensive projections; trophic support more feasible
Habenula	Epithalamus adjacent to third ventricle; lateral and medial divisions	Negative outcome processing; promotes withdrawal from failed strategies	May process persistent threats and failures	SIGNIFICANT: Hyperactivity inhibits dopamine/ serotonin; mediates learned helplessness; anti-reward processing	Increased metabolic activity	Hyperactivity in depression; excessive negative prediction error signaling; monoamine suppression	Potential DBS target (experimental); ketamine may reduce habenula hyperactivity	: Small but critical structure; reducing hyperactivity may be therapeutic; inhibitory modulation preferable

Brain Structure	Location/ Anatomy	Role in Stress	Role in Anxiety	Role in Depression	Structural Changes	Functional Changes	Management Targets	Stem Cell Potential
Basal Ganglia	Striatum (caudate, putamen), globus pallidus, substantia nigra	Motor and motivational effects of stress; habit formation during chronic stress	Altered habit learning; may contribute to compulsive behaviors in some anxiety disorders	Psychomotor symptoms (retardation or agitation); reduced motivation; anhedonia (via ventral striatum)	Volume reductions in caudate; altered striatal connectivity	Reduced striatal responses to rewards; altered habit learning; reduced goal-directed behavior	Dopaminergic medications variable efficacy; behavioral activation; ECT affects basal ganglia function	Ventral striatum (NAc) higher priority; dorsal striatum less clear target; connectivity restoration important
Cerebellum	Posterior fossa; cortex and deep nuclei	Implicated in emotional processing beyond motor functions; may modulate stress responses	Emerging evidence for anxiety-related processing	Consistently shows structural and functional abnormalities in depression	Volume reductions in vermal and hemispheric regions	Altered connectivity with frontal cortex; possible role in cognitive symptoms	Indirect target; cerebellar TMS experimental; most treatments don't specifically target cerebellum	Complex structure; roles in mood unclear; not primary target currently

NSCs Prefrontal Cortex

The prefrontal cortex occupies the anterior portion of the frontal lobes, comprising approximately 30% of total cortical volume in humans. This region demonstrates the most dramatic evolutionary expansion in primates and particularly humans, reflecting its roles in higher-order cognitive functions.

Major subdivisions include:

- **Dorsolateral prefrontal cortex (dlPFC)**: Located on the lateral surface of the frontal lobes, this region supports working memory, cognitive flexibility, planning, and abstract reasoning.
- **Ventromedial prefrontal cortex (vmPFC)**: Located on the medial and orbital surfaces, this region integrates emotional and cognitive information, supports value-based decision-making, and regulates autonomic and endocrine responses.
- **Anterior cingulate cortex (ACC)**: Positioned in the medial frontal lobe surrounding the corpus callosum, the ACC divides into dorsal (cognitive) and ventral (affective) subregions. The dorsal ACC supports conflict monitoring, error detection, and cognitive control. The ventral/pregenual/subgenual ACC (areas 24, 25, 32) regulates emotional processing and autonomic function.
- **Orbitofrontal cortex (OFC)**: Located above the orbits of the eyes, the OFC processes reward and punishment information, supports value representations, and guides goal-directed behavior.

The prefrontal cortex serves as the brain's executive control system, implementing top-down regulation of subcortical structures, including the amygdala, hippocampus, and hypothalamus. It enables conscious regulation of emotional responses, inhibition of prepotent responses, flexible updating of behavioral strategies based on changing circumstances, and maintenance of goals in working memory despite distractions. The vmPFC and ACC exert inhibitory control over amygdala reactivity, implementing emotion regulation strategies such as cognitive reappraisal (reinterpreting emotional situations to alter their impact). The dlPFC supports cognitive strategies for managing stress and maintaining goal-directed behavior despite emotional interference. The prefrontal cortex demonstrates protracted maturation, continuing development into the mid-twenties. This extended developmental timeline creates a vulnerability window during adolescence and early adulthood when subcortical emotional systems have matured but prefrontal regulatory systems remain developing. The structure also shows particular sensitivity to stress effects, with acute stress impairing prefrontal function while enhancing amygdala responses, creating a neurobiological basis for emotion dysregulation under stress.

PFC NSCs may support the neural systems that allow humans to regulate emotions using reflection, planning, and executive control. Because the PFC interacts with limbic structures, such as the amygdala, having regenerative potential in this area may help maintain top-down emotional regulation, particularly under stress.

Cognitive impairments—including reduced attention and decreased problem-solving ability—are commonly documented in prolonged stress and depressive conditions. PFC NSCs might aid in maintaining the health of networks responsible for decision-making and coping strategies. This could reduce vulnerability to maladaptive responses.

In anxiety disorders, inadequate prefrontal inhibition of fear circuits can result in excessive worry or avoidance. NSCs located in the PFC may assist in supporting neural pathways needed to calm overactive threat responses. Their plasticity-related functions might help individuals regain more balanced emotional control.

Reduced prefrontal neurogenesis has been associated with increased rumination and anhedonia in mood disorders. By potentially supporting neural resilience, PFC NSCs could help preserve motivation, social engagement, and behavioral activation. These elements are considered central to functional recovery in depressive states.

The prefrontal cortex (PFC) exerts top-down regulation over limbic structures. NSCs in this region could provide ongoing support for the maintenance of cognitive control over emotions. Potential advantages include:

- Stress: Enhancing coping strategies and reducing maladaptive responses
- Anxiety: Improving regulation of fear circuits and reducing intrusive worry

- Depression: Sustaining motivation, decision-making, and behavioral engagement

Preserved PFC neurogenesis may reduce vulnerability to rumination and impaired emotional regulation.

Hypothalamic NSCs

The hypothalamus is a small but critical structure located below the thalamus at the base of the brain, forming the floor and walls of the third ventricle. Despite comprising less than 1% of brain volume, it contains numerous distinct nuclei organized into medial and lateral zones and anterior (supraoptic), middle (tuberal), and posterior (mammillary) regions.

Key nuclei relevant to stress, anxiety, and depression include:

- **Paraventricular nucleus (PVN)**: Contains neurons producing corticotropin-releasing hormone (CRH), the initiating signal of the HPA axis stress response. These neurons also produce vasopressin, which potentiates CRH effects.
- **Suprachiasmatic nucleus (SCN)**: The brain's master circadian pacemaker, receiving direct input from the retina and coordinating circadian rhythms throughout the body.
- **Arcuate nucleus**: Contains neurons regulating appetite, energy balance, and reward, relevant to appetite and weight changes in depression.
- **Preoptic area**: Regulates sleep-wake cycles and body temperature.

The hypothalamus serves as the primary integration center linking the nervous system and endocrine system, coordinating physiological responses to stress, emotion, and changing environmental conditions. It regulates fundamental survival functions, including food intake, water balance, body temperature, sleep-wake cycles, circadian rhythms, and reproductive behavior. In stress responses, PVN neurons detect threatening stimuli through inputs from the amygdala, hippocampus, and brainstem, and initiate the HPA axis cascade by releasing CRH into the hypophyseal portal system. The hypothalamus also activates sympathetic nervous system responses through projections to the brainstem and spinal autonomic centers. Disruption of hypothalamic function contributes to the neurovegetative symptoms characteristic of depression: altered appetite and weight, sleep disturbances, circadian rhythm abnormalities, and reduced libido. The hypothalamus receives negative feedback from circulating cortisol, which should terminate stress responses once threats pass, but this feedback mechanism often becomes impaired in chronic stress and depression.

Hypothalamic NSCs may assist in sustaining circuits that control the body's endocrine and autonomic stress responses. Because the hypothalamus initiates the HPA axis, which regulates cortisol and other stress hormones, NSCs in this region could help maintain balanced stress signaling. This balance may be relevant for resilience under persistent psychological strain.

Disturbances in sleep, appetite, and metabolic function are frequently observed in depression and anxiety. Hypothalamic NSCs might aid in supporting the cellular health of systems regulating these biological rhythms. Modulating these functions may indirectly contribute to emotional stability and stress recovery.

Some experimental studies suggest that these NSCs may protect against HPA axis overactivation, a common consequence of prolonged stress exposure. Their presence may be associated with the brain's ability to return to baseline after a stressor. This potential regulation might reduce physiological anxiety manifestations such as tension and elevated heart rate.

Neural adaptability in the hypothalamus can influence overall emotional well-being by linking brain activity with bodily feedback. Hypothalamic NSCs might contribute to maintaining this integration. Through such mechanisms, they may have a theoretical role in preventing the progression of stress responses into clinical anxiety or depressive disorders.

Hypothalamic NSCs may assist in maintaining the integrity of circuits regulating the hypothalamic–pituitary–adrenal (HPA) axis. Through neuroendocrine coordination, they might influence:

- Stress: Balanced cortisol release and recovery after stress activation
- Anxiety: Regulation of autonomic physiological arousal (heart rate, tension)

- Depression: Maintenance of sleep–wake cycles and appetite patterns, which are often disturbed

Experimental models suggest NSCs in this region may help prevent excessive HPA axis activation, a hallmark in chronic stress and depression.

NSCs of the Pituitary Gland

The pituitary gland, often called the "master gland," is a pea-sized endocrine structure located in the sella turcica (a bony cavity at the base of the skull) and connected to the hypothalamus by the pituitary stalk (infundibulum). It comprises two distinct portions with different embryological origins: the anterior pituitary (adenohypophysis) and the posterior pituitary (neurohypophysis). The anterior pituitary develops from oral ectoderm and contains multiple cell types secreting different hormones. The posterior pituitary consists of axon terminals from hypothalamic neurons and stores/releases hormones synthesized in the hypothalamus.

The anterior pituitary serves as a critical intermediary in the HPA axis, translating hypothalamic CRH signals into systemic endocrine responses. Corticotroph cells in the anterior pituitary express CRH receptors; when CRH binds these receptors, corticotrophs synthesize and release adrenocorticotropic hormone (ACTH) into the bloodstream. ACTH travels through circulation to the adrenal glands, where it stimulates cortisol synthesis and release. This cascade amplifies hypothalamic signals, converting neural information into hormonal messages that coordinate body-wide stress responses. The anterior pituitary also releases other hormones relevant to mood and stress, including thyroid-stimulating hormone (hypothyroidism is associated with hypothyroidism, and prolactin. The pituitary demonstrates plasticity in response to chronic stress. Repeated CRH stimulation can alter corticotroph sensitivity, contributing to HPA axis dysregulation in chronic stress and psychiatric disorders. The gland is also subject to negative feedback from cortisol, which inhibits ACTH release when cortisol levels are sufficient—a feedback mechanism often impaired in depression.

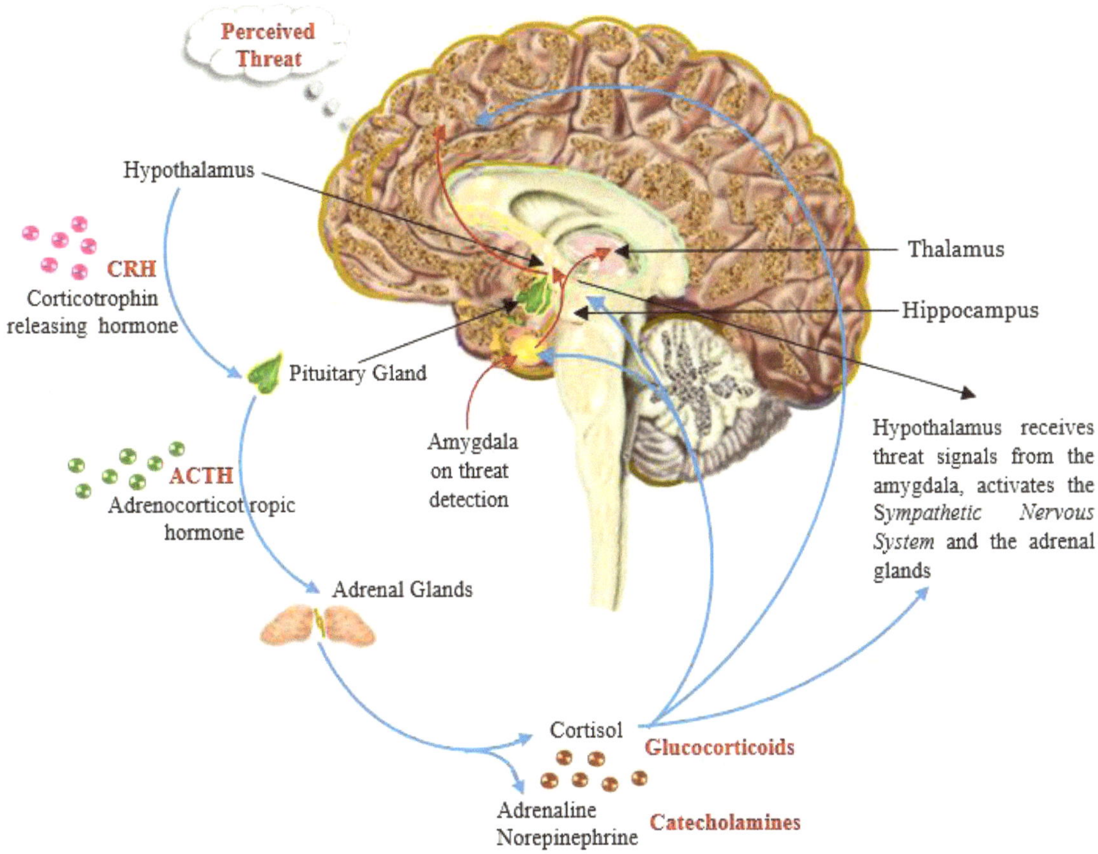

A schematic illustration of the brain's complex circuitry mediating fear responses and anxiety behavior along with hormonal mechanisms responsible for hyperactivity of the HPA axis in response to a threat.

Source: Lleuvelyn A. Cacha, Roman R. Poznanski, Sheikh Hussain Salleh, Ahmad Zubaidi Abdul Latif, Tengku M. Ariff. Anxiety-related circuitry in affective neuroscience. J. Mol. Clin. Med. 2020, 3(3), 67–74.

NSCs of the Pituitary Gland may support ongoing hormonal adaptability throughout life. Because the pituitary regulates key stress-associated hormones, including adrenocorticotropic hormone (ACTH), the observations suggest that NSCs in this region can influence neuroendocrine responsiveness. Their ability to generate new endocrine cells may provide structural support for hormonal recalibration in response to chronic stress exposure.

The scientific studies propose that pituitary NSCs can contribute to better resilience in hypothalamic–pituitary–adrenal (HPA) axis signaling. Since HPA axis dysregulation is frequently reported in stress-related and depressive disorders, NSCs renewing hormone-secreting cells could potentially assist in normalizing cortisol production patterns. This could help stabilize daily stress-recovery cycles, though such mechanisms remain under active investigation.

Research models indicate that pituitary plasticity may mediate improvements in mood and energy regulation. Dysfunction in pituitary hormone output - including growth hormone, prolactin, and thyroid-related hormones - has been associated with depressive symptoms such as fatigue, anhedonia, and cognitive slowing. NSC-driven pituitary remodeling, therefore, may be explored for supportive prospects in endocrine-linked depression.

In anxiety-related conditions, enhanced pituitary adaptability might reduce exaggerated HPA stress reactivity. If NSCs can support finer hormonal control, the escalation of physiological anxiety responses (e.g., heightened cortisol, rapid autonomic arousal) may be tempered. These ideas highlight a biologically plausible connection between pituitary NSCs and emotional regulation.

NSCs Frontal lobe - The Anterior Cingulate Cortex

The anterior cingulate cortex (ACC) forms the frontal portion of the cingulate gyrus, a band of cortex surrounding the corpus callosum in the medial frontal lobe. The ACC is typically divided into dorsal cognitive (dACC) and ventral affective (vACC) subdivisions based on anatomical connectivity and functional specialization. The dorsal ACC (areas 24' and 32') maintains connections with lateral prefrontal cortex, parietal cortex, and motor systems, positioning it to monitor cognitive processes and guide behavioral adjustments. The ventral ACC, particularly the pregenual and subgenual regions (areas 24, 25, 32), connects extensively with the amygdala, hippocampus, hypothalamus, nucleus accumbens, and other limbic structures, enabling integration of emotional, cognitive, and autonomic information.

The dorsal ACC functions as a conflict monitoring system, detecting situations where multiple response options compete or when errors occur. It signals the need for increased cognitive control, recruiting lateral prefrontal regions to resolve conflicts and adjust behavior. This region activates during tasks requiring error monitoring, pain processing, effortful attention, and response selection. The ventral/ subgenual ACC plays crucial roles in emotion regulation, autonomic control, and motivation. Area 25 (subgenual ACC) shows consistent abnormalities in depression, with elevated metabolic activity in depressed states that normalizes with successful management. This region regulates emotional responses, modulates autonomic function, and influences reward processing. The ACC demonstrates altered function across stress-related disorders. In depression, the subgenual ACC shows hyperactivity correlating with rumination and negative mood. In anxiety disorders, the ACC shows heightened responses to errors and conflict, potentially reflecting excessive performance monitoring and worry. Deep brain stimulation of area 25 has shown promise for treatment-resistant depression, highlighting the region's causal role in mood regulation.

NSCs of the frontal lobe region engaged in emotional monitoring, conflict detection, and regulation of negative affect. It is revealed that NSCs–driven plasticity in the ACC may support adaptive decision-making and error processing, especially under emotionally challenging circumstances.

The ACC is frequently implicated in anxiety and depressive disorders, where structural and functional disruptions are commonly documented. NSCs of the frontal lobe region may assist in preserving cognitive control functions that help individuals shift attention away from distressing thoughts or exaggerated threat interpretations. This is particularly relevant for generalized anxiety and rumination-based depression.

Some studies propose that NSC-supported cellular renewal may contribute to strengthened connectivity with other emotional regulation areas, including the prefrontal cortex and limbic structures. Improvements in these circuits may enhance coping responses, emotional flexibility, and motivation during stress.

In stress-response models, ACC-related neurogenesis may reduce excessive activation of the HPA axis by promoting more efficient cognitive reinterpretation of stressful stimuli. While still theoretical, NSC involvement in this region could represent a target for future therapies aimed at improving top-down emotional regulation in mood and anxiety disorders.

NSCs Forebrain - The Nucleus Accumbens and Ventral Striatum

The nucleus accumbens (NAc) is located in the ventral striatum at the junction between the caudate nucleus and putamen. It comprises two subregions: the core (more similar to dorsal striatum) and the shell (more closely connected with the extended amygdala). The NAc receives convergent inputs from the prefrontal cortex, amygdala, hippocampus, and ventral tegmental area (VTA), positioning it to integrate information about rewards, emotions, contexts, and motivational states. The ventral tegmental area, located in the midbrain, contains dopamine neurons that project to the nucleus accumbens, prefrontal cortex, and other forebrain regions. This mesolimbic dopamine pathway forms the core of the brain's reward system.

The nucleus accumbens mediates motivated behavior, translating reward-related information into action. Dopamine release in the NAc signals reward prediction errors (when outcomes differ from expectations), motivating approach behavior toward reward-associated stimuli and learning about action-outcome contingencies. The NAc shell particularly contributes to processing reward hedonic value (the pleasure derived from rewards) and integrating emotional and contextual information to guide behavior. The core supports action selection and vigor, translating motivational states into behavioral output. In the context of mood disorders, the NAc demonstrates critical involvement in anhedonia—the inability to experience pleasure from previously rewarding activities, a cardinal symptom of depression. Depressed individuals show reduced NAc activation to rewarding stimuli, decreased dopamine signaling, and diminished motivation for reward pursuit. This reward circuitry dysfunction explains the lack of enjoyment, reduced motivation, and behavioral withdrawal characteristic of depression. Chronic stress reduces dopamine signaling in the mesolimbic pathway and induces structural changes in NAc neurons, creating a neurobiological substrate for stress-induced anhedonia and depression vulnerability. The NAc also contributes to social reward processing; social anhedonia and withdrawal in depression reflect dysfunction in these circuits.

NAc and ventral striatum are key components of the brain's reward and motivation system. Emerging evidence indicates that NSCs or progenitor of these structures can influence dopamine-dependent reward processing and behavioral reinforcement. Their regenerative potential may support healthy engagement with pleasurable activities.

In depressive disorders characterized by anhedonia (reduced ability to experience pleasure), NSCs in these reward centers may help counteract motivational deficits by promoting neural circuit rejuvenation. Animal models have shown that enhancing cellular plasticity in the NAc can improve social interaction and reward-seeking behaviors, suggesting possible translational pathways.

Chronic stress is known to impair dopaminergic signaling in the ventral striatum. The NSCs mechanisms might help restore balance by generating new neurons or enhancing synaptic remodeling. This could theoretically improve resilience against stress-induced emotional blunting and loss of interest.

For anxiety disorders, reward circuit NSCs may aid in shifting behavioral patterns away from avoidance and toward exploration and positive learning. While the research is still emerging, the possibility exists that neurogenic support in these regions may reduce maladaptive negative prediction biases, helping restore motivation and overall emotional well-being.

NSCs Cerebral cortex - The Insula

The insula is a cortical region buried within the lateral sulcus, hidden beneath the frontal, parietal, and temporal opercula. It connects extensively with limbic structures (amygdala, anterior cingulate), sensory cortices, and autonomic control regions. The insula demonstrates a posterior-to-anterior gradient, with posterior regions processing basic interoceptive information and anterior regions integrating this information with emotional and cognitive content.

The insula serves as the brain's interoceptive cortex, representing bodily physiological states including heartbeat, respiration, gastrointestinal sensations, pain, temperature, and visceral sensations. This interoceptive awareness provides the foundation for subjective emotional feelings; the anterior insula particularly integrates bodily sensations with emotional significance, contributing to conscious emotional experience. In anxiety disorders, the insula shows heightened activity, potentially reflecting amplified awareness of bodily arousal sensations (racing heart, breathlessness, trembling) that characterize anxiety states. In panic disorder, the insula's hyperactivation may contribute to catastrophic interpretation of bodily sensations—misinterpreting normal variations in heartbeat or breathing as signs of imminent medical catastrophe. The insula also processes disgust, uncertainty, and anticipatory anxiety. Its dysfunction contributes to the hypervigilance toward bodily sensations in anxiety disorders and the somatic symptoms often prominent in depression (fatigue, pain, gastrointestinal complaints).

NSCs of the Cerebral Cortex may support the maintenance of brain networks involved in internal bodily awareness and emotional perception. The insula processes interoceptive cues such as changes in heart rate or breathing that often accompany stress responses, so NSC-driven plasticity could help preserve balanced interpretation of these signals. Enhanced adaptability here might reduce misinterpretation of normal bodily sensations as threatening, a characteristic frequently seen in panic and anxiety disorders.

Studies suggest that insular function impacts the integration of emotional and social context with physiological states. NSCs of the Cerebral Cortex may contribute to sustaining circuits that evaluate the emotional meaning of discomfort or stress. This could potentially reduce the escalation of distress into maladaptive fear responses under chronic anxiety conditions.

In depressive disorders, reduced insula volume and connectivity have been reported. As such the new neuron formation and synaptic remodeling supported by NSCs of the Cerebral Cortex might help restore functional integration between the insula and limbic-prefrontal networks. This could be linked to improved emotion-body coherence, which plays a role in mood stabilization.

The insula is also part of the salience network, determining which external or internal cues deserve attention. NSC-related plasticity may assist in adjusting attentional biases—shifting them away from persistent negative internal focus, thereby offering benefits in both stress-induced hypervigilance and depressive rumination.

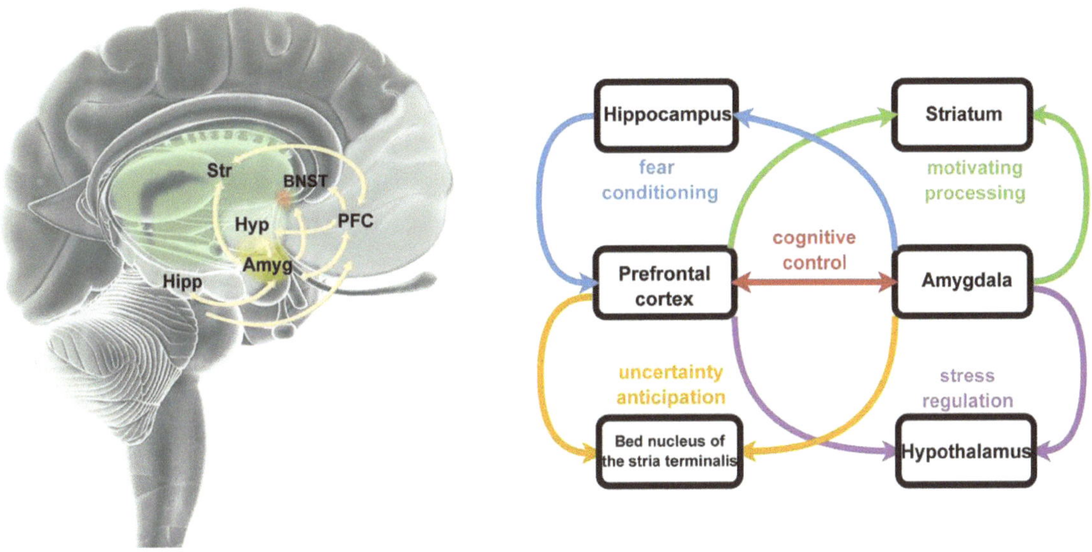

Schematic presentation of anxiety-related functional systems and brain structures. The arrows indicate the neural projections between two brain regions. The pathological interactions of the six critical regions in the anxiety network bring about functional abnormality for patients with anxiety disorders. Amyg, Amygdala; BNST, Bed nucleus of the stria terminalis; Hipp, Hippocampus; Hyp, Hypothalamus; PFC, Prefrontal cortex; Str, Striatum.

Source: Xie S, Zhang X, Cheng W, Yang Z. Adolescent anxiety disorders and the developing brain: comparing neuroimaging findings in adolescents and adults. General Psychiatry. 2021;34:e100411.

NSCs Thalamus

The thalamus comprises two egg-shaped masses of gray matter flanking the third ventricle in the diencephalon. It contains numerous distinct nuclei organized into functional groups: specific relay nuclei (transmitting sensory and motor information to the cortex), association nuclei (connecting with association cortices), and non-specific nuclei (modulating cortical arousal). The mediodorsal nucleus connects extensively with the prefrontal cortex and limbic structures. The anterior nuclei connect with the hippocampus and cingulate cortex, participating in memory circuits. The intralaminar nuclei modulate arousal and attention.

The thalamus serves as the brain's primary relay station, processing and transmitting sensory information (except olfaction) to cortical regions. It filters sensory information based on behavioral relevance and arousal state, functioning as a gatekeeper determining which information reaches conscious awareness. In stress and anxiety, the thalamus transmits threat-related sensory information to both cortical regions (enabling conscious perception) and the amygdala (enabling rapid threat response). The thalamus also modulates arousal and attention, with hyperactivation contributing to the heightened vigilance and sensory sensitivity characteristic of anxiety disorders. In depression, thalamic connectivity with prefrontal and limbic regions becomes disrupted, potentially contributing to cognitive and emotional symptoms. Some neuroimaging studies report reduced thalamic volumes in chronic depression.

The thalamus acts as a central sensory relay hub, directing information toward emotional and cognitive areas. NSC of the thalamus may support continuous refinement of sensory gating, which is crucial for distinguishing threatening from non-threatening stimuli. The thalamic NSCs plasticity is associated with improved sensory modulation under stress.

Thalamic circuits are strongly connected with the amygdala and prefrontal cortex, forming pathways deeply involved in anxiety regulation. NSCs may strengthen the ability of these pathways to adapt, potentially helping limit hypersensitive emotional reactivity to mild or ambiguous cues.

In depression, altered thalamo-cortical connectivity is commonly observed, contributing to impaired cognitive processing and reduced attention to rewarding experiences. Neurogenic processes initiated by NSCs of the thalamus may help maintain balanced signal transmission, enhancing the brain's capacity to process positive sensory information.

Thalamic dysfunction is also linked to sleep disturbances—a major comorbidity in stress-related disorders. Because NSCs of the thalamus could influence rhythm-related neuronal populations, they may contribute to stabilization of sleep–wake patterns, indirectly supporting emotional health.

NSCs Brainstem - The Locus Coeruleus

The locus coeruleus (LC) is a small brainstem nucleus located in the dorsal pons near the fourth ventricle. Despite containing only approximately 15,000-30,000 neurons per hemisphere in humans, these neurons project throughout the entire neuraxis, innervating virtually all brain regions through extensive axonal arborization.

The LC contains the brain's primary noradrenergic neurons, serving as the major source of norepinephrine in the central nervous system. LC neurons fire in two modes: tonic baseline activity maintaining optimal arousal and attention, and phasic bursts in response to salient stimuli, particularly threats or unexpected important events. LC activation produces widespread brain arousal, enhances sensory processing, promotes vigilance, facilitates memory consolidation for important events, and coordinates the body's stress response by activating sympathetic nervous system. The LC contributes to the fight-or-flight response and regulates the sleep-wake cycle. In anxiety disorders, the LC shows hyperactivity, contributing to excessive arousal, hypervigilance, and exaggerated startle responses. In depression, LC function may become dysregulated, with some individuals showing excessive activity (anxious depression, agitation) and others showing hypoactivity (psychomotor retardation, fatigue). The LC's noradrenergic projections are targets of antidepressant medications, particularly serotonin-norepinephrine reuptake inhibitors (SNRIs).

LC of the brainstem is essential for arousal, vigilance, and stress mobilization. Experimental evidence suggests that LC NSCs may help maintain noradrenergic neuron populations across the lifespan. This could preserve the capacity for flexible alertness rather than chronic hyperarousal, a key feature of anxiety disorders.

Under prolonged stress, LC neurons can become overactive, amplifying fear circuitry and negative anticipation. NSC-related mechanisms may help restore more adaptive firing patterns, potentially reducing exaggerated startle responses and physiological anxiety.

In depression, disrupted norepinephrine signaling contributes to diminished motivation, concentration difficulties, and fatigue. LC NSCs have the ability to support the recovery of noradrenergic pathways that encourage engagement with the environment and cognitive efficiency.

Additionally, the LC regulates autonomic responses, including cardiovascular and respiratory adjustments under stress. Neural renewal in this region may help buffer the body against prolonged physiological strain that contributes to chronic stress pathology.

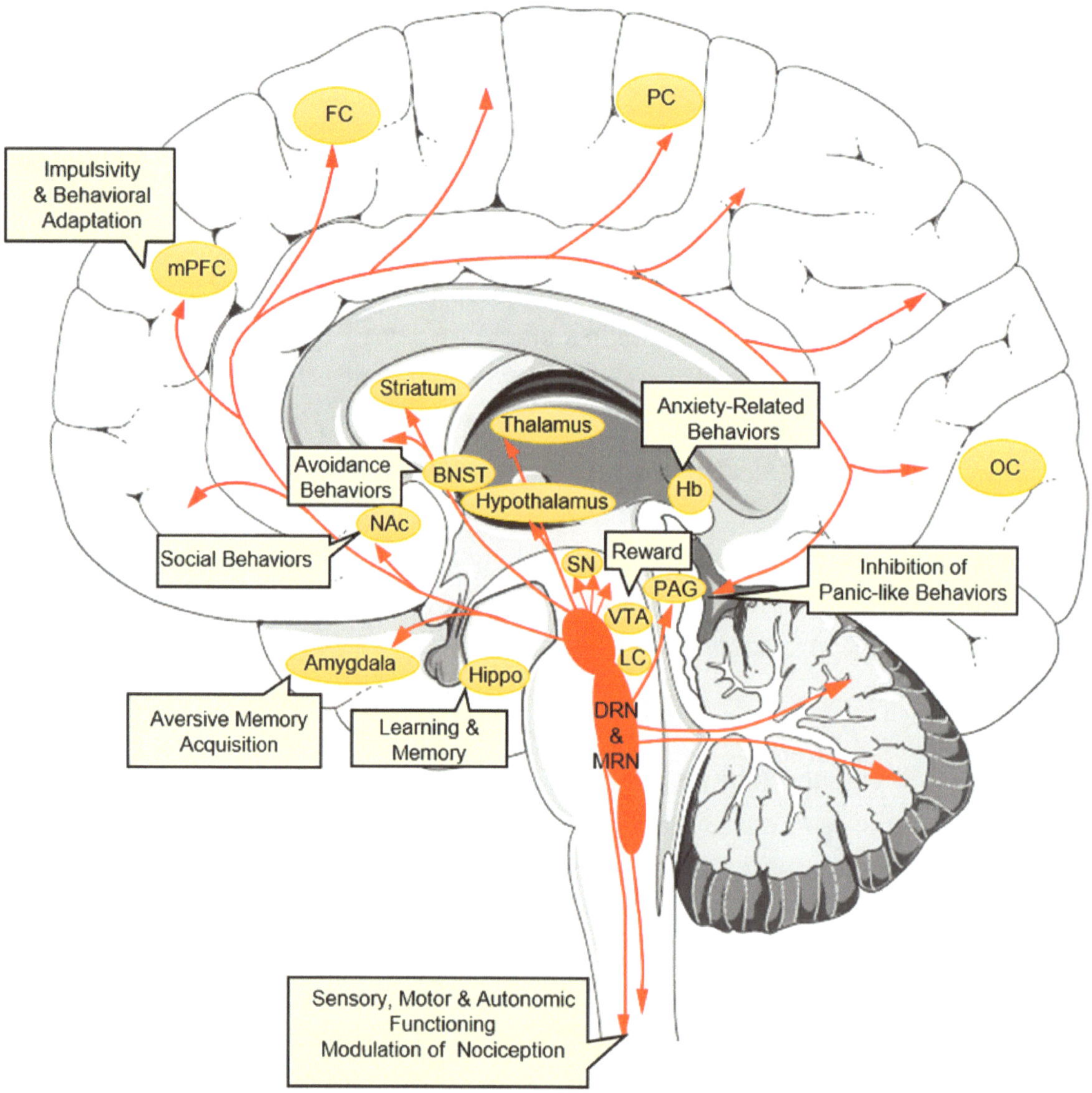

Serotonergic Pathways. In addition to the dorsal and median raphe nuclear complex, many serotonergic neurons are found in the reticular region of the lower brain stem, which is subdivided into caudal and rostral groups. Serotonergic neurons of the rostral system (caudal linear, dorsal raphe, and median raphe nuclei) mostly terminate in the dorsal and medial

raphe nuclei, which in turn innervate much of the rest of the CNS by diffuse projections. Serotonergic neurons of the caudal group (raphe magnus, raphe obscurus, raphe pallidus nuclei) descend into the brain stem and the spinal cord along the dorsal horn, ventral horn motor nuclei and thoracic cord intermediolateral column and are mostly involved in sensory, motor and autonomic functioning. The central gray matter and the ependyma of the central canal also receives 5-HT input in a pattern of 5-HT nerve plexus. Serotonergic signaling regulates impulsivity and behavioral adaptation through actions within the medial prefrontal cortex (mPFC). Serotonergic innervation is present throughout the NAc and involved in social behaviors. Moreover, serotonergic fibers innervate the amygdala and enhance aversive memory acquisition. Signaling of 5-HT in the periaqueductal gray (PAG) is involved in behavioral inhibition and prevent panic-like behaviors. Additionally, serotonergic innervation is present throughout the bed nucleus of the stria terminalis (BNST) and could promote or inhibit approach and avoidance behaviors. The expression of the fear- and anxiety-related defensive behavioral responses of the habenula (Hb) is also regulated by serotonergic projections. The presence of 5-HT has been observed in the pons, medulla, septal area and specific areas of the thalamus, hypothalamus, substantia nigra (SN) and locus coeruleus (LC). The hippocampus (Hippo), the suprachiasmatic nucleus, the olfactory bulb and the medial septum nucleus receive 5-HT innervation from the MRN. Likewise, serotonergic fibers are one of the afferent fibers innervating and affecting the activity of cerebellar circuitry (Dölen 2015; Jorgensen 2007; Puig and Gulledge 2011; Linley et al. 2017; Saitow et al. 2012)

Source: Poorhamze, Mahsa & Moravej, Fahimeh & Arabi, Mehrnoosh & Shahriari, Elahe & Mehrabi, Soraya & Ward, Richard & Ahadi, Reza & Joghataei, Mohammad Taghi. (2022). The Roles of Serotonin in Neuropsychiatric Disorders. Cellular and Molecular Neurobiology. 42.

NSCs Brainstem - The Raphe Nuclei

The raphe nuclei comprise a chain of midline nuclei extending through the brainstem from the midbrain to the medulla. They are divided into rostral (midbrain and pontine) and caudal (medullary) groups. The dorsal and median raphe nuclei in the rostral group contain the majority of serotonergic neurons and project widely throughout the forebrain.

The raphe nuclei contain the brain's principal serotonergic neurons, serving as the primary source of serotonin (5-HT) throughout the central nervous system. Serotonin modulates diverse functions, including mood, anxiety, sleep, appetite, pain perception, impulsivity, and social behavior. Different serotonin receptor subtypes (at least 14 identified) mediate varied effects in different brain regions. Serotonergic projections to the prefrontal cortex influence executive function and emotion regulation. Projections to the amygdala and hippocampus modulate emotional reactivity and memory. Projections to the hypothalamus affect appetite, sleep, and neuroendocrine function. Serotonergic dysfunction represents a central feature of depression and anxiety pathophysiology, forming the basis for selective serotonin reuptake inhibitor (SSRI) antidepressants. Reduced serotonin synthesis, altered receptor sensitivity, and impaired serotonergic neurotransmission contribute to mood and anxiety symptoms. The raphe nuclei themselves show reduced volume and neuronal counts in post-mortem studies of individuals who died by suicide.

NSCs of the Raphe Nuclei of the Brainstem in this region may support the replenishment and preservation of serotonergic neurons. It is known that neurogenesis here can enhance adaptive stress coping and social behavior.

Serotonin imbalances are widely associated with anxiety and depression. By maintaining flexibility in the serotonin system, raphe NSCs may help reduce excessive fear signaling and emotional dysregulation. This could be particularly relevant for disorders involving heightened worry or persistent negative mood.

Chronic stress can impair serotonergic neurons and reduce synaptic plasticity. NSCs may assist in countering these effects by providing new cells or strengthening synaptic networks, potentially supporting more effective mood regulation mechanisms.

Because serotonin also modulates pain perception and sleep—both often disrupted in anxiety and depression—neurogenic support in the raphe nuclei may indirectly contribute to reduced stress burden and improved overall functioning.

NSCs Forebrain - The Bed Nucleus of the Stria Terminalis

The bed nucleus of the stria terminalis (BNST) is a small structure located in the basal forebrain, forming part of the extended amygdala along with the central nucleus of the amygdala and portions of the nucleus accumbens shell. The BNST receives inputs from the amygdala, hippocampus, and prefrontal cortex, and projects to the hypothalamus, brainstem autonomic centers, and ventral tegmental area.

The BNST mediates sustained anxiety and vigilance in response to uncertain, unpredictable, or temporally distant threats—distinct from the amygdala's role in immediate fear responses. While the amygdala responds rapidly to acute threats, the BNST sustains anxious states over extended periods, maintaining hypervigilance and physiological arousal when threats are ambiguous or context-dependent. The BNST activates the HPA axis and autonomic nervous system, producing the sustained physiological arousal characteristic of anxiety disorders. It processes contextual information about threat probability and maintains anxiety during prolonged uncertainty. The BNST's role in sustained anxiety makes it particularly relevant to generalized anxiety disorder, where chronic worry about uncertain future threats predominates. CRH signaling within the BNST promotes anxiety-like behaviors in animal models, and the structure shows altered function in human anxiety disorders. The BNST also contributes to negative affective states during drug withdrawal, linking stress and addiction systems.

NSCs of the Forebrain in this region may support neural remodeling that helps distinguish between probable and remote dangers. This could moderate prolonged worry states that characterize generalized anxiety disorder.

The research indicates that BNST hyperactivity is associated with chronic stress exposure. NSCs of the Forebrain - related adaptability may support dampening of stress-induced neuronal sensitization, reducing persistent fear of diffuse, non-specific threats.

The BNST interacts with the HPA axis through stress-hormone regulation pathways. By maintaining healthy connectivity and neuronal populations, NSCs may help normalize stress hormone release, potentially decreasing both anxiety and depressive symptoms associated with HPA dysregulation.

Additionally, because the BNST contributes to social behavioral responses under stress, NSC-mediated plasticity might support better social engagement and reduction of stress-linked avoidance patterns.

NSCs Midbrain - The Periaqueductal Gray

The periaqueductal gray (PAG) surrounds the cerebral aqueduct in the midbrain, organized into dorsal, lateral, and ventrolateral columns with distinct connectivity and functions. The PAG receives inputs from the amygdala, prefrontal cortex, and hypothalamus, and projects to brainstem nuclei controlling defensive behaviors, autonomic responses, and pain modulation.

The PAG coordinates defensive behavioral responses to threats, organizing different defensive strategies based on threat imminence and type. The dorsal PAG mediates active defensive responses (fight-or-flight), while the ventrolateral PAG mediates passive defensive responses (freezing, quiescence). The PAG also controls pain perception through descending pain modulation pathways. In panic disorder, PAG dysfunction may contribute to panic attacks—sudden surges of fear and physiological arousal resembling responses to immediate threats. The PAG can trigger panic-like responses when activated, and imaging studies show PAG activation during panic attacks in humans. The structure may represent a "suffocation alarm system," with abnormal PAG sensitivity contributing to panic attacks characterized by breathlessness and choking sensations. The PAG's pain modulation functions relate to the high comorbidity between chronic pain and depression/anxiety. Altered PAG function may contribute to both increased pain sensitivity and emotional disturbance in these comorbid conditions.

NSCs' Midbrain, including the Periaqueductal Gray, may support fine-tuning of these responses, preventing excessive fear reactions and maladaptive fight-or-flight activation. This could be especially relevant in panic and trauma-related anxiety disorders.

Neural adaptability in the PAG might contribute to balanced endogenous analgesia, reducing the somatic distress that frequently accompanies chronic stress and depression. Experimental models demonstrate that PAG plasticity can influence the perception of pain or stress.

The PAG also interacts with emotional memory circuits. NSCs may help update fear associations, enabling individuals to gradually adjust defensive reactions when a threat is no longer present.

Because PAG hyperactivation is often linked to overwhelming anxiety responses, the NSCs Midbrain might support shifts toward more measured and adaptive behavioral patterns under stress.

NSCs Epithalamus - The Habenula

The habenula is a small epithalamic structure located adjacent to the third ventricle, comprising lateral and medial subnuclei. The lateral habenula receives inputs from basal ganglia, limbic regions, and prefrontal cortex, and projects to midbrain monoaminergic nuclei, including the raphe (serotonin), ventral tegmental area (dopamine), and locus coeruleus (norepinephrine).

The lateral habenula functions as an "anti-reward" center, activating in response to disappointing outcomes, punishment, and failure. It inhibits midbrain dopamine and serotonin neurons, reducing motivation and positive affect. The habenula processes negative prediction errors (when outcomes are worse than expected) and promotes behavioral withdrawal and inhibition. In depression, the habenula shows hyperactivity, excessively inhibiting monoaminergic systems and contributing to anhedonia, reduced motivation, and negative bias in processing outcomes. The structure may mediate learned helplessness—the passive behavioral response that develops after repeated uncontrollable aversive experiences, a key animal model of depression. The habenula represents an emerging target for deep brain stimulation in treatment-resistant depression, with preliminary evidence suggesting that modulating habenular activity can improve depressive symptoms.

NSCs Epithalamus, including the Habenula, support changes of aversion-related circuits, potentially reducing negative behavioral biases.

AT the same time, the habenular neurogenesis can influence dopamine and serotonin outputs through connections with midbrain monoaminergic systems. This suggests possible relevance to both depressive symptoms and anxiety-related fear generalization.

Under chronic stress, habenular circuits can become increasingly sensitive to negative outcomes. NSC-driven flexibility may allow recalibration it, helping restore emotional responses that reflect real-world conditions rather than excessive negativity.

According to that, the habenula plays a role in circadian regulation via pineal interactions, and maintaining its plasticity may support normalized sleep and daily mood cycling, which are often dysregulated in major depressive and anxious states.

Nano-peptides

Neuropeptides are small protein-like molecules of nano size used by brain cells to communicate. They modulate emotional behavior, stress responses, and mood regulation with high specificity. Unlike traditional neurotransmitters, neuropeptides have longer-lasting effects, influence multiple signaling pathways, and often produce more targeted therapeutic outcomes. These characteristics make them promising therapeutic targets for improving stress responses, reducing anxiety, and alleviating depression.

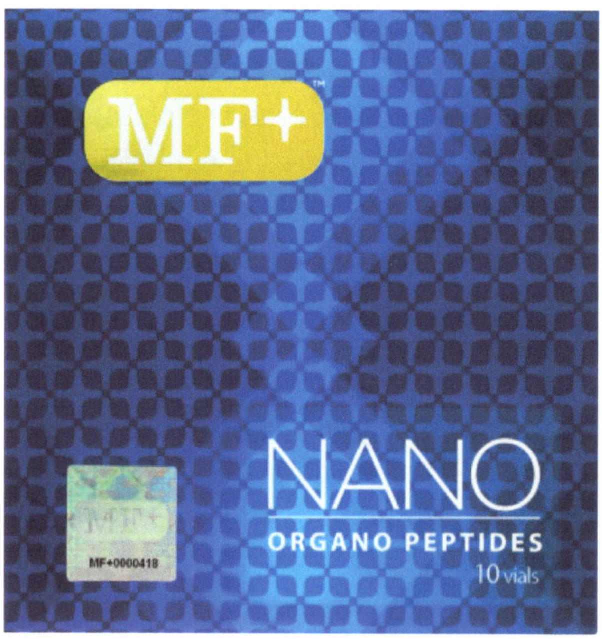

Source: (Product courtesy Stellar BioMolecular Research, Germany).

Amygdala Neuropeptides

The amygdala regulates fear processing, emotional memory, and threat detection.

Key advantages:

- Precision in modulating fear circuits ĸeduces hyper-reactivity seen in anxiety and trauma disorders.
- Regulation of stress signaling to the hypothalamus pelps normalize the stress hormone cascade.
- Enhanced emotional resilience - NPY and oxytocin promote calmness, bonding, and adaptive fear extinction.
- Reduced excessive threat interpretation improves responses to non-dangerous stimuli often misread as threats.

These mechanisms support the prevention of amygdala overactivation, a hallmark in anxiety and traumatic stress conditions.

Hypothalamus Neuropeptides

The hypothalamus governs the HPA axis, autonomic responses, sleep, and appetite.

Advantages:

- Direct control over cortisol and systemic stress hormones
- Restoration of sleep–wake balance through orexin system modulation
- Improved autonomic stability → reduced heart rate, muscle tension, and panic-like physiological responses
- Enhanced mood through endocrine–neural integration, bridging brain and body regulation

Optimal hypothalamic neuropeptide signaling is crucial for preventing long-term stress toxicity.

Hippocampus-Related Neuropeptides

The hippocampus supports memory formation, cognitive flexibility, and contextual interpretation of stress.

Advantages:

- Promotion of neurogenesis and synaptic plasticity - helps reverse brain atrophy seen in chronic stress and depression.
- Reduction of reactive cortisol damage to memory structures
- Better memory-based fear discrimination - avoids generalized anxiety from harmless cues.
- Cognitive support during mood recovery, improving concentration and decision-making.

Prefrontal Cortex Neuropeptides

The prefrontal cortex (PFC) regulates executive control, emotional inhibition, and resilience.

Advantages:

- Stronger emotional regulation over limbic structures (especially the amygdala)
- Improvement in attention and decision-making impaired by anxiety and depression
- Increased stress tolerance and coping behaviors
- Reduction of impulsivity and maladaptive responses
- Healthy PFC neuropeptide activity restores top-down regulation of overwhelming emotional states.

Combined Benefits Across Brain Structures

Benefit	Amygdala	Hypothalamus	Hippocampus	PFC
Fear Reduction	✓	—	✓	✓
Mood Stability	✓	✓	✓	✓
Cortisol Regulation	✓	✓	✓	—
Cognitive Resilience	—	—	✓	✓
Autonomic Balance	—	✓	—	✓
Neuroplastic Recovery	—	✓	✓	✓

Neuropeptides provide unique clinical value because they:

- Act on entire neural networks, not only single synapses
- Work in harmony with hormones, immune signals, and neurotransmitters
- Offer long-acting neuromodulation with less frequent dosing needs
- Support repair and recovery rather than only symptom suppression
- Can be delivered via nanocarriers, intranasal routes, or targeted therapies
- Represent a pathway toward personalized mental health approach

Nano peptides of transfer factor

Chronic stress is known to activate the immune system and promote a pro-inflammatory state. When exposure to stressors is prolonged, elevated cytokines such as interleukin-6 (IL-6), tumor necrosis factor-alpha (TNF-α), and C-reactive protein (CRP) may cross or signal across the blood–brain barrier and influence neuronal function. This immune-driven process forms the basis of the "cytokine hypothesis" of mood disorders, suggesting that excessive inflammation may alter neurotransmission, neuroplasticity, and hypothalamic–pituitary–adrenal (HPA) axis regulation. As a result, experimental strategies targeting immune dysregulation have been considered in the context of stress-related anxiety and depression.

INTEGRATED PATHOPHYSIOLOGY (a)

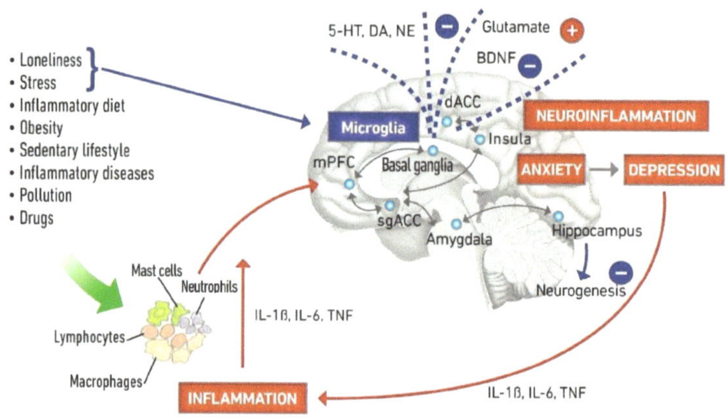

INTEGRATED TREATMENT (b)

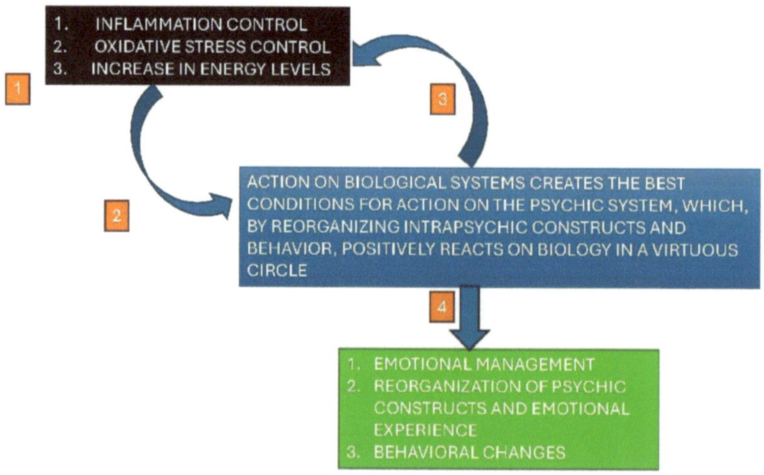

Source: Bottaccioli AG, Bologna M, Bottaccioli F. Rethinking Depression—Beyond Neurotransmitters: An Integrated Psychoneuroendocrineimmunology Framework for Depression's Pathophysiology and Tailored Treatment. International Journal of Molecular Sciences. 2025; 26(6):2759.

Nano-peptide transfer factors—small immunologically active peptides derived from immune cells and delivered using nanocarrier technology—may offer potential advantages in this area. Their nanoscale formulation can improve transport efficiency, stability, and cellular uptake, allowing targeted interaction with immune receptors. These peptides may help moderate excessive inflammatory signaling by supporting balanced immune responses rather than broad suppression. Experimental studies suggest that nano-transfer factors could influence the regulation of T-cells, normalization of cytokine levels, and reduction of neuroinflammation that contributes to altered emotional states.

In the context of stress, nano-peptide transfer factors may assist in preventing prolonged inflammatory responses that can impair neural circuits involved in resilience and emotional coping. By potentially stabilizing inflammatory biomarkers such as IL-6, TNF-α, and CRP, these peptides could help reduce the negative feedback on mood-regulating systems including serotonin, dopamine, and glutamate pathways. This might lead to better preservation of neuroplasticity within brain regions like the hippocampus and prefrontal cortex, which are often vulnerable to stress-induced structural changes.

Regarding anxiety disorders, immune modulation mediated through nano-peptide transfer factors may contribute to reducing heightened autonomic reactivity and excessive amygdala responsiveness to perceived threats. As chronic low-grade inflammation has been associated with persistent worry and hypervigilance, mitigation of neuroimmune disturbances could support more adaptive emotional processing.

In depressive conditions, where inflammation-driven anhedonia and fatigue are common, immune-supportive nano-transfer peptides may help restore healthier communication between immune and neural systems. By promoting more normalized cytokine activity, these peptides could improve neurotransmitter synthesis and energy metabolism, factors influencing motivation and mood regulation. Their small size and engineered delivery systems may enable deeper access into neuroimmune interfaces that are otherwise difficult for conventional therapies to reach.

Overall, nano-peptide transfer factors may represent a promising direction for integrative approaches that combine immune modulation with mental health management. Their potential role in addressing inflammation-linked emotional disorders is still under ongoing scientific exploration, but early findings suggest they may help counter biological pathways through which chronic stress contributes to anxiety and depression.

Mito-organells

Mitochondria, the cellular organelles producing energy through oxidative phosphorylation, show dysfunction in stress-related psychiatric disorders. Given the brain's enormous energy demands—consuming 20% of the body's energy despite representing only 2% of body weight—mitochondrial dysfunction profoundly affects neural function.

Energy metabolism impairment.

Multiple studies demonstrate reduced brain glucose metabolism in depression, particularly in the prefrontal cortex, anterior cingulate cortex, and other regions. Positron emission tomography using fluorodeoxyglucose (FDG-PET) consistently shows hypometabolism in these regions, correlating with symptom severity. This reduced metabolism partly reflects decreased neuronal activity, but also may indicate primary mitochondrial dysfunction that impairs energy production.

Post-mortem studies reveal altered expression of mitochondrial genes and proteins in depression. Genes encoding electron transport chain components, ATP synthase subunits, and other mitochondrial proteins show reduced expression. Mitochondrial DNA copy number, reflecting mitochondrial abundance, decreases in peripheral blood cells of depressed individuals, potentially indicating systemic mitochondrial dysfunction.

The consequences of impaired energy metabolism are wide-ranging. Neurons require enormous ATP supplies to maintain membrane potentials, support neurotransmitter synthesis and release, and power active transport. Insufficient ATP compromises all these functions. Synaptic transmission is particularly energy-intensive, and mitochondrial dysfunction disproportionately affects synaptic regions where energy demands are highest.

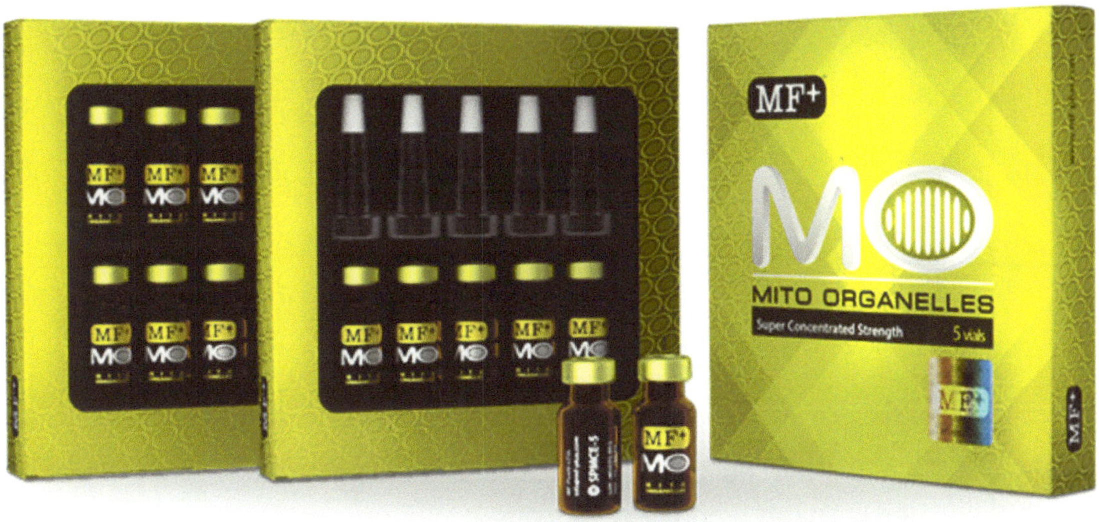

Source: (Product courtesy Stellar BioMolecular Research, Germany).

Oxidative stress.

Mitochondria are both producers and targets of reactive oxygen species (ROS). During normal oxidative phosphorylation, electrons occasionally leak from the electron transport chain, reacting with oxygen to produce superoxide and other ROS. Cells possess antioxidant defenses (superoxide dismutase, glutathione peroxidase, catalase) that normally neutralize ROS, but when ROS production exceeds antioxidant capacity, oxidative stress results.

Depression and chronic stress are associated with elevated oxidative stress, as evidenced by increased lipid peroxidation products, oxidative DNA damage, and protein oxidation. Antioxidant defenses become depleted—glutathione levels decrease, and antioxidant enzyme activities reduce. This oxidative damage affects all cellular components but particularly damages mitochondria themselves, creating a vicious cycle where mitochondrial dysfunction produces ROS that further damages mitochondria.

Oxidative stress has multiple deleterious effects. It damages proteins, inactivating enzymes and disrupting cellular functions. Lipid peroxidation damages cell membranes, particularly affecting neurons, where membrane integrity is critical for electrical signaling. Oxidative DNA damage can cause mutations and impair gene expression. Oxidative modification of neurotransmitter receptors and transporters disrupts neurotransmission.

Calcium dysregulation.

Mitochondria play critical roles in buffering intracellular calcium, taking up calcium when cytosolic levels rise excessively and releasing it when more calcium signaling is needed. In depression and stress conditions, this mitochondrial calcium buffering becomes impaired. Mitochondria become calcium-overloaded, which impairs their respiratory function and can trigger apoptosis (programmed cell death) through opening of the mitochondrial permeability transition pore.

Dysregulated calcium signaling has wide-ranging consequences for neuronal function. Calcium serves as a ubiquitous second messenger regulating neurotransmitter release, gene expression, synaptic plasticity, and numerous other processes. Impaired calcium homeostasis thus disrupts many aspects of neuronal function. Excessive intracellular calcium activates degradative enzymes, including calpains and phospholipases, that damage cellular structures.

Mitochondrial dynamics alterations.

Mitochondria are dynamic organelles that continuously undergo fission (division into smaller mitochondria) and fusion (combining to form larger mitochondrial networks). This dynamic balance maintains a healthy mitochondrial population, with fission allowing removal of damaged mitochondria through mitophagy (selective autophagy of mitochondria) while fusion allows mitochondria to share contents and complement each other's deficiencies.

In depression and chronic stress, mitochondrial dynamics become dysregulated. Some studies report increased fission, producing fragmented mitochondrial networks with impaired function. Proteins regulating mitochondrial dynamics (dynamin-related protein 1/Drp1 for fission; mitofusins and OPA1 for fusion) show altered expression and activity. Impaired mitophagy allows the accumulation of dysfunctional mitochondria that should have been eliminated.

The subcellular distribution of mitochondria also becomes disrupted. Neurons require mitochondria at specific locations—particularly at synapses where energy demands are highest, but mitochondrial transport along axons and dendrites becomes impaired in stress conditions. This means that synapses lack adequate energy supplies, even if the total number of mitochondria is preserved.

Mitochondrial interactions with stress pathways.

Mitochondria interact bidirectionally with cellular stress responses. Glucocorticoids affect mitochondrial function directly through receptors on mitochondrial membranes and indirectly through regulating nuclear gene expression of mitochondrial proteins. Excessive glucocorticoid exposure impairs mitochondrial respiration, increases ROS production, and sensitizes cells to apoptosis.

Mitochondria also regulate HPA axis function. Mitochondrial dysfunction in hypothalamic neurons affects their capacity to respond appropriately to feedback signals, potentially contributing to HPA axis dysregulation. The bidirectional relationship between mitochondria and stress hormones creates potential vicious cycles where stress impairs mitochondrial function, mitochondrial dysfunction affects stress system regulation, and dysregulated stress responses further damage mitochondria.

Inflammatory cytokines impair mitochondrial function through multiple mechanisms. TNF-α and other cytokines disrupt the electron transport chain, increase ROS production, and sensitize mitochondria to calcium-induced permeability transition. This provides a mechanistic link between neuroinflammation and energy metabolism deficits in depression.

Therapeutic implications

Recognition of mitochondrial dysfunction suggests potential intervention approaches. Compounds supporting mitochondrial function—coenzyme Q10, L-carnitine, creatine, nicotinamide riboside (NAD+ precursor)—show promise in depression, though evidence remains preliminary. Antioxidants targeting mitochondria specifically (MitoQ, SkQ1) represent novel experimental approaches. Exercise, which powerfully stimulates mitochondrial biogenesis (production of new mitochondria), may partly exert antidepressant effects through improving mitochondrial function.

Some antidepressant medications demonstrate mitochondrial protective effects independent of their neurotransmitter effects. SSRIs can reduce oxidative stress, improve mitochondrial respiration, and protect against mitochondrial-mediated apoptosis. Whether these mitochondrial effects contribute to clinical efficacy or merely represent epiphenomena remains unclear.

The need for mito-organells of mitochondria

Mitochondria are essential cellular organelles responsible for producing energy through ATP, regulating oxidative balance, and supporting healthy cell survival. Because brain tissue has a very high energy demand, optimal mitochondrial function is crucial for maintaining stable emotional, cognitive, and stress-regulatory processes. Growing evidence shows that disruptions in mitochondrial activity contribute significantly to the development and progression of stress-related, anxiety-related, and depressive disorders.

Mitochondria are major regulators of the hypothalamic–pituitary–adrenal (HPA) axis, the system that controls the body's reaction to stress. When mitochondria function efficiently, stress hormones such as cortisol are released in a controlled manner, allowing quick adaptation to challenges. However, mitochondrial dysfunction can create excessive or prolonged cortisol exposure, leading to mood changes, impaired memory, and anxiety symptoms. Supporting mitochondrial health, therefore, helps maintain a balanced stress response.

Another advantage of healthy mitochondria is their role in oxidative stress control. During chronic psychological stress, the production of harmful free radicals increases, damaging neurons and synapses. Mitochondria with strong antioxidant defenses help protect brain cells from inflammation and degeneration. This protection is vital for brain regions involved in emotional regulation, such as the amygdala, hippocampus, and prefrontal cortex.

Mitochondria also influence the production of important neurotransmitters, including serotonin, dopamine, and GABA. These chemical messengers are central to mood stability, anxiety management, and motivation. When mitochondrial metabolism is optimal, neurotransmitter synthesis is supported, improving emotional balance and cognitive functioning. Conversely, mitochondrial impairment is commonly observed in depression and anxiety disorders.

Finally, mitochondria play a key role in neuroplasticity, the brain's ability to adapt, recover, and form new connections. Neuronal growth factors such as BDNF (Brain-Derived Neurotrophic Factor) depend heavily on mitochondrial energy production. Strong mitochondrial performance enhances memory, learning, resilience to stress, and response to treatment. Therapeutic strategies that boost mitochondrial efficiency—including targeted nutrients, lifestyle interventions, and emerging mitochondrial-based medical therapies—show promise in reducing symptoms and restoring brain health.

Chapter 8

Physiotherapy in the Management of Borderline mental disorders (stress, anxiety, depression)

Transcranial Direct Current Stimulation (tDCS)

Introduction to Transcranial Direct Current Stimulation

Transcranial direct current stimulation represents a non-invasive neuromodulation technique that involves applying weak electrical currents to the scalp to modulate cortical excitability and neural activity. Unlike other brain stimulation methods such as electroconvulsive therapy or transcranial magnetic stimulation, tDCS delivers low-intensity direct current, typically ranging from 0.5 to 2 milliamperes, through electrodes placed on specific scalp locations corresponding to targeted brain regions. The technique has gained considerable research interest as a potential intervention for various psychiatric conditions, including major depressive disorder, anxiety disorders, and stress-related conditions.

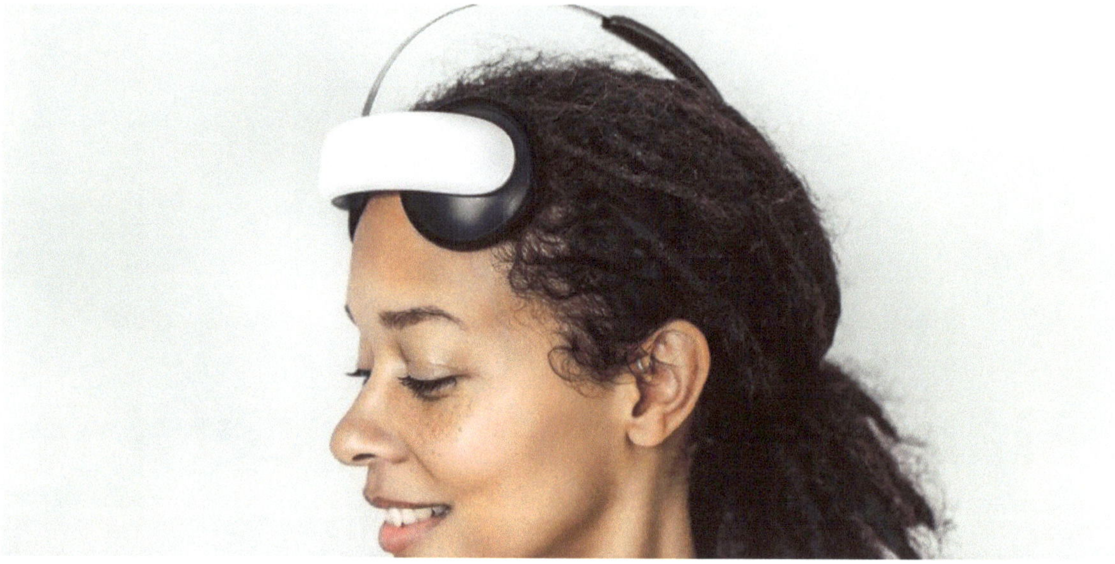

Source: European Wellness

The fundamental principle underlying tDCS involves the modulation of neuronal membrane potentials through application of weak electrical fields. When direct current passes through brain tissue, it creates electrical fields that can influence the resting membrane potential of cortical neurons. Anodal stimulation, where the positive electrode (anode) is placed over the target region, generally increases cortical excitability by depolarizing neuronal membranes, making neurons more likely to fire action potentials. Conversely, cathodal stimulation, where the negative electrode (cathode) is positioned over the target area, typically reduces cortical excitability through hyperpolarization, making neurons less likely to reach firing threshold.

However, the effects of tDCS extend beyond simple modulation of neuronal excitability during stimulation. Research has demonstrated that tDCS can induce neuroplastic changes that persist beyond the stimulation period, potentially offering lasting therapeutic benefits. These aftereffects appear to involve mechanisms similar to long-term potentiation and long-term depression—fundamental processes underlying learning and memory. The duration and magnitude of aftereffects depend on various parameters, including current intensity, stimulation duration, electrode montage, and individual subject characteristics.

The appeal of tDCS as a potential intervention approach stems from several characteristics: it is non-invasive and painless when properly administered, it demonstrates a favorable safety profile in research studies, the equipment is relatively inexpensive compared to other neuromodulation technologies, it can be combined with other interventions such as cognitive training or psychotherapy, and it may offer a home-based option for some applications. These features have prompted extensive investigation into tDCS applications for psychiatric conditions, though important questions regarding optimal protocols, mechanisms of action, and long-term efficacy remain under investigation.

Neurobiological Mechanisms of Action

Immediate Effects on Cortical Excitability

The immediate effects of tDCS on cortical activity have been characterized through various neurophysiological measurement techniques. Transcranial magnetic stimulation studies examining motor evoked potentials have demonstrated that anodal tDCS over the motor cortex increases cortical excitability, evidenced by larger motor evoked potentials, while cathodal stimulation produces the opposite effect. These changes occur during stimulation and can persist for minutes to hours afterward, depending on stimulation parameters.

Electroencephalography studies have revealed that tDCS modulates oscillatory brain activity across various frequency bands. Anodal stimulation may increase power in higher frequency bands associated with cortical activation, while cathodal stimulation may enhance lower frequency activity associated with cortical inhibition. These oscillatory changes correlate with behavioral and cognitive effects of stimulation, suggesting that modulation of neural synchrony and network dynamics contributes to tDCS effects.

Functional magnetic resonance imaging investigations have shown that tDCS affects not only activity in regions directly beneath electrodes but also in connected brain regions, indicating that tDCS influences distributed neural networks. For example, stimulation of the dorsolateral prefrontal cortex produces changes in limbic regions including the amygdala and hippocampus, despite these structures being anatomically distant from the stimulation site. This network-level modulation may be particularly relevant for psychiatric applications, where dysfunction involves circuits spanning multiple brain regions.

Neuroplastic Mechanisms

The lasting effects of tDCS appear to involve neuroplastic mechanisms similar to those underlying learning and memory. Research in animal models and human studies suggests several potential mechanisms through which tDCS may induce enduring changes in brain function.

Synaptic plasticity modifications represent a primary mechanism. Studies have indicated that tDCS can modulate long-term potentiation and long-term depression, fundamental processes involving activity-dependent strengthening or weakening of synaptic connections. The polarity-dependent effects of tDCS—anodal stimulation facilitating LTP-like plasticity and cathodal stimulation promoting LTD-like changes—suggest that tDCS can bias synaptic modification processes in specific directions.

The role of NMDA receptors in tDCS effects has been demonstrated through pharmacological studies. Administration of NMDA receptor antagonists blocks the aftereffects of tDCS, suggesting that glutamatergic neurotransmission through NMDA receptors is necessary for inducing lasting changes. This parallels the well-established role of NMDA receptors in various forms of synaptic plasticity. The calcium influx through NMDA receptors triggered by tDCS-induced depolarization may initiate intracellular signaling cascades leading to gene expression changes and structural synaptic modifications.

GABAergic neurotransmission also appears to contribute to tDCS effects. Studies using magnetic resonance spectroscopy to measure GABA concentrations have found that tDCS can alter cortical GABA levels, with effects varying based on stimulation polarity and parameters. Given GABA's role in regulating cortical excitability and in various psychiatric conditions, modulation of GABAergic function may contribute to therapeutic effects.

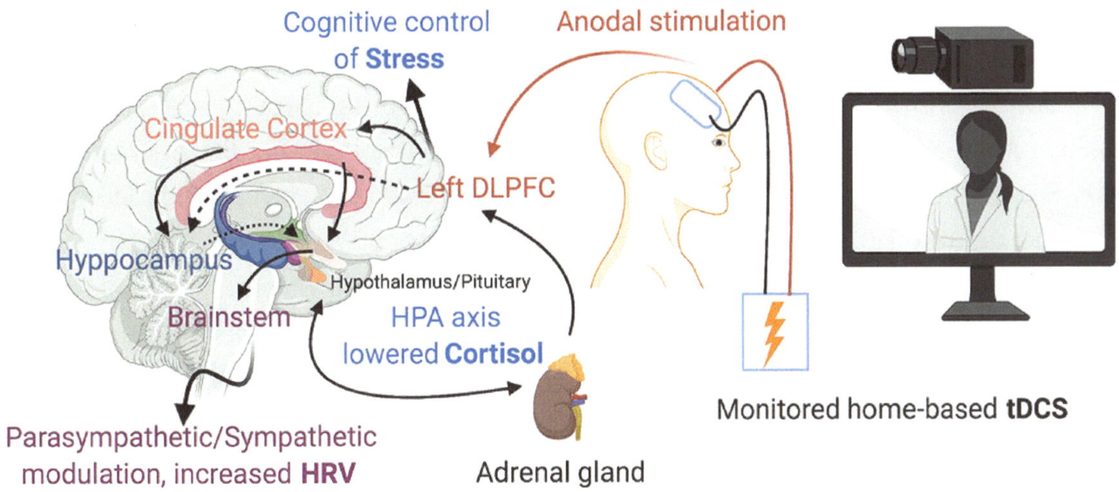

Home-based tDCS over the left DLPFC promoting the cognitive control of Stress, changes in the HPA axis and Parasympathetic/Sympathetic modulation. Created with BioRender.com.

Source: Castelo-Branco L and Fregni F (2020) Home-Based Transcranial Direct Current Stimulation (tDCS) to Prevent and Treat Symptoms Related to Stress: A Potential Tool to Remediate the Behavioral Consequences of the COVID-19 Isolation Measures? Front. Integr. Neurosci. 14:46.

Modulation of neurotrophic factors represents another potential mechanism through which tDCS may promote lasting changes. Animal studies have suggested that electrical stimulation can increase expression of brain-derived neurotrophic factor, a key molecule supporting neuronal survival, synaptic plasticity, and neurogenesis. While direct evidence in humans remains limited, the possibility that tDCS enhances neurotrophic support could explain some of its potential therapeutic effects, particularly given the well-documented reductions in BDNF associated with depression and chronic stress.

Changes in neurotransmitter systems beyond glutamate and GABA have been investigated. Positron emission tomography studies have examined tDCS effects on dopaminergic, serotonergic, and other neurotransmitter systems, with some evidence suggesting that stimulation can influence neurotransmitter release and receptor binding. However, findings remain preliminary and require replication.

Effects on Neural Networks and Connectivity

Beyond local effects on stimulated cortical regions, tDCS appears to modulate functional connectivity within and between brain networks. Resting-state functional MRI studies examining spontaneous brain activity patterns have demonstrated that tDCS can alter connectivity in several networks relevant to psychiatric disorders.

The default mode network, which shows hyperactivity and altered connectivity in depression, may be modulated by tDCS targeting prefrontal regions. Some studies have reported that prefrontal tDCS can normalize default mode network connectivity patterns, potentially reducing rumination and excessive self-focused thought characteristic of depression. However, findings vary across studies, and the optimal parameters for achieving desired connectivity changes remain under investigation.

Fronto-limbic connectivity, frequently disrupted in mood and anxiety disorders, represents another target of tDCS effects. Stimulation of prefrontal cortex has been shown to influence amygdala reactivity and prefrontal-amygdala functional connectivity, potentially enhancing top-down regulatory control over emotional processing. This mechanism could be particularly relevant for anxiety disorders and emotional dysregulation in depression.

The salience network, involved in detecting behaviorally relevant stimuli and switching between other networks, shows alterations in anxiety and depression. Some research suggests that tDCS may normalize salience network function, though this remains an area requiring further investigation.

Task-based functional connectivity studies, examining brain network interactions during specific cognitive or emotional tasks, have provided evidence that tDCS can enhance task-relevant network engagement and suppress task-irrelevant network activity. This suggests that tDCS may improve the efficiency of neural processing, potentially contributing to cognitive and emotional benefits.

Modulation of Inflammatory Processes

Emerging evidence suggests that tDCS may influence neuroinflammatory processes, which have been increasingly recognized as contributing to depression and potentially anxiety disorders. Animal studies have indicated that electrical stimulation can reduce pro-inflammatory cytokine expression while increasing anti-inflammatory mediators. In humans, some small studies have reported changes in peripheral inflammatory markers following tDCS protocols, though findings remain preliminary and require replication in larger samples.

The mechanisms through which tDCS might affect inflammation are not fully understood but could involve several pathways. Direct effects on glial cells, including microglia and astrocytes, represent one possibility. Modulation of the autonomic nervous system balance, shifting from sympathetic toward parasympathetic tone, could reduce inflammatory signaling. Effects on the hypothalamic-pituitary-adrenal axis might influence stress hormone levels and their downstream effects on immune function.

If confirmed, the anti-inflammatory effects of tDCS could be particularly relevant for the inflammatory subtype of depression, which shows elevated inflammatory markers and may respond differently to conventional interventions. However, this remains a speculative application that requires substantial additional research before clinical implementation can be considered.

Technical Parameters and Protocols

Electrode Montages

The spatial arrangement of electrodes, referred to as the montage, critically determines which brain regions are affected by tDCS and the nature of the effects. Various montages have been investigated for psychiatric applications, with selection based on hypotheses about which brain regions and circuits are dysfunctional in specific conditions.

For depression, the most extensively studied montage involves anodal stimulation of the left dorsolateral prefrontal cortex with the cathode typically positioned over the right supraorbital region (above the right eye). This montage aims to increase activity in left prefrontal regions that show hypoactivity in depression while potentially reducing right-sided hyperactivity. The left dorsolateral prefrontal cortex is involved in executive function, working memory, and emotion regulation—functions frequently impaired in depression.

Alternative montages for depression have positioned the cathode over the right dorsolateral prefrontal cortex, creating a bifrontal montage that may enhance laterality effects. Some protocols have targeted the ventromedial prefrontal cortex, important for emotion regulation and extinction learning, though stimulating deeper structures like vmPFC poses challenges given that tDCS primarily affects superficial cortical regions.

For anxiety disorders, montages targeting prefrontal regulatory regions and potentially modulating amygdala activity have been explored. Anodal stimulation of the left dorsolateral prefrontal cortex, similar to depression protocols, has been investigated based on prefrontal hypoactivation in anxiety. Some research has examined right-sided stimulation or bilateral montages, given the complex laterality of anxiety-related processing.

High-definition tDCS, which uses multiple smaller electrodes to create more focal stimulation fields, represents a technical advancement allowing more precise targeting. This approach may reduce current spread to non-target regions and enable stimulation of smaller, more specific cortical areas. However, high-definition tDCS requires more complex equipment and has been less extensively studied than conventional tDCS in psychiatric applications.

Stimulation Parameters

Current intensity in most psychiatric tDCS studies has ranged from 1 to 2 milliamperes. Lower intensities may be insufficient to produce robust effects, while higher intensities increase the risk of adverse effects and may not necessarily enhance benefits. Some research has explored whether 2 mA produces superior outcomes compared to 1 mA, with mixed results suggesting that simply increasing intensity may not be optimal and that individual differences in brain anatomy, physiology, and genetics may influence optimal intensity.

Stimulation duration per session has typically ranged from 20 to 30 minutes in psychiatric research. Shorter durations may produce limited effects, while durations beyond 30 minutes do not clearly enhance benefits and may increase discomfort. The relationship between stimulation duration and aftereffect duration is nonlinear—longer stimulation sessions do not necessarily produce proportionally longer-lasting effects, and very long sessions might even produce paradoxical effects or homeostatic regulatory responses that limit benefits.

The number of sessions and treatment course duration vary considerably across studies. Protocols have ranged from single sessions used for acute effects to extended courses involving daily sessions over several weeks. For depression, many studies have employed protocols of 10 to 20 sessions administered daily or five times weekly over two to four weeks, paralleling typical courses of antidepressant medications or repetitive transcranial magnetic stimulation. Whether longer treatment courses enhance outcomes or whether there may be optimal treatment durations beyond which benefits plateau remains under investigation.

Session frequency represents another parameter under investigation. Daily sessions have been most common, but some research has explored twice-daily sessions or sessions administered on alternate days. The optimal interval between sessions likely depends on how long stimulation effects persist and on homeostatic mechanisms that may limit the cumulative effects of closely-spaced sessions.

Application to Depressive Disorder

The application of tDCS to major depressive disorder has been the most extensively investigated psychiatric use of this technology. Multiple randomized controlled trials have examined tDCS efficacy for depression, with meta-analyses attempting to synthesize findings across studies.

Early pilot studies and small randomized trials suggested that active tDCS targeting left dorsolateral prefrontal cortex might produce antidepressant effects superior to sham stimulation. These studies typically employed protocols involving 10 to 20 sessions over two to four weeks, using 1 to 2 mA current intensity for 20 to 30 minutes per session. Participants often showed modest symptom improvements on standardized depression scales, with some studies reporting response rates comparable to antidepressant medications in head-to-head comparisons.

However, larger multi-center trials have produced mixed results. Some have replicated positive findings, demonstrating significant antidepressant effects of active compared to sham stimulation. Others have found no significant differences between active and sham conditions, despite adequate power to detect clinically meaningful effects. This inconsistency has generated considerable debate about tDCS efficacy for depression.

Meta-analyses combining results across multiple trials have generally concluded that active tDCS produces statistically significant antidepressant effects compared to sham stimulation, with standardized mean differences in the small to medium range. However, several considerations temper enthusiasm. First, effect sizes are generally smaller than those for established interventions such as antidepressant medications or electroconvulsive therapy. Second, substantial heterogeneity exists across studies, suggesting that effects may vary considerably depending on population characteristics, stimulation parameters, or other factors. Third, publication bias remains a concern, as studies showing positive results may be more likely to be published than those finding null results.

Treatment-resistant depression has been a particular focus, given limited options for individuals who do not respond to conventional interventions. Some studies have specifically examined tDCS in treatment-resistant populations, with mixed results. While some individuals with treatment-resistant depression may benefit from tDCS, response rates appear lower than in less treatment-resistant samples, and many treatment-resistant patients show minimal improvement.

Long-term outcomes following tDCS for depression remain inadequately characterized. Most studies have focused on acute effects during and immediately after treatment courses, with limited follow-up data. The few studies examining outcomes weeks to months after tDCS cessation have reported high relapse rates, suggesting that acute benefits may not persist without maintenance strategies. Some research has explored maintenance tDCS protocols involving periodic booster sessions, with preliminary evidence suggesting such approaches might help sustain improvements, though systematic investigation is needed.

Application to Anxiety Disorders

Research examining tDCS for generalized anxiety disorder remains relatively limited compared to depression studies. GAD involves chronic worry, hypervigilance, and autonomic arousal, with neurobiological models implicating hypoactive prefrontal regulatory regions and hyperactive threat-detection systems including the amygdala and bed nucleus of the stria terminalis.

The rationale for tDCS in GAD parallels that for depression—enhancing prefrontal cortex activity might improve top-down control over excessive worry and threat-vigilant processing. Anodal stimulation of the dorsolateral prefrontal cortex, the most commonly studied montage for GAD, aims to strengthen cognitive control and reduce involuntary worry processes.

Small pilot studies have explored tDCS for GAD with mixed results. Some have reported reductions in anxiety symptoms following multi-session tDCS protocols, while others have found minimal effects. The limited number of studies, small sample sizes, and methodological variations preclude firm conclusions about efficacy.

One challenge in GAD research relates to measuring outcomes. Anxiety symptoms fluctuate considerably, and distinguishing treatment effects from natural fluctuation or placebo responses requires adequate sample sizes and rigorous methodology. Additionally, GAD often involves chronic symptoms persisting for years, and whether brief tDCS interventions can produce lasting changes in such chronic conditions remains questionable.

Combining tDCS with cognitive-behavioral therapy for GAD represents a conceptually appealing approach. CBT for GAD involves learning to recognize and modify worry processes, develop distress tolerance, and implement worry management strategies—learning that might theoretically be enhanced by tDCS-induced prefrontal plasticity. However, research specifically examining tDCS-CBT combinations for GAD is minimal.

Application to Chronic Stress

Transcranial direct current stimulation offers several potential advantages as an approach for managing chronic stress, supported by preliminary research evidence. The non-invasive nature of tDCS represents a primary advantage, as the technique delivers weak electrical currents through scalp electrodes without requiring surgical procedures, anesthesia, or significant disruption to daily activities. This contrasts with more invasive neuromodulation approaches such as vagus nerve stimulation or deep brain stimulation, making tDCS more acceptable to individuals seeking stress management interventions. The technique demonstrates a favorable safety profile in research studies, with adverse effects typically limited to mild, transient sensations such as tingling beneath electrodes or occasional mild headaches that resolve shortly after stimulation cessation, representing a considerable advantage over pharmacological approaches that may produce systemic side effects including weight gain, sexual dysfunction, or metabolic disturbances. The relatively brief duration of individual sessions, typically 20 to 30 minutes, enhances practical feasibility for individuals with demanding schedules who contribute to elevated stress levels. Research examining acute stress responses has provided some evidence supporting tDCS benefits, with studies reporting that anodal stimulation targeting dorsolateral prefrontal cortex may attenuate cortisol responses to laboratory stressors and reduce subjective anxiety during stress exposure, suggesting direct modulation of hypothalamic-pituitary-adrenal axis reactivity. Preliminary investigations in occupationally stressed populations have reported improvements in perceived stress, sleep quality, and cognitive performance following multi-session tDCS protocols, though these findings require replication in adequately controlled trials. The potential for combining tDCS with established stress management approaches represents another advantage, as stimulation-enhanced neuroplasticity might theoretically facilitate learning and implementation of coping strategies taught in cognitive-behavioral stress management, mindfulness-based interventions, or other psychological approaches, creating synergistic benefits. The relatively low cost of tDCS equipment compared to other neuromodulation technologies such as repetitive transcranial magnetic stimulation may enhance accessibility if efficacy is established, though current costs still exceed many individuals' means. Research suggesting that tDCS can modulate prefrontal-limbic connectivity patterns indicates potential for addressing circuit-level dysfunction underlying maladaptive stress responses, with neuroimaging studies demonstrating that prefrontal stimulation influences amygdala reactivity and enhances regulatory control over emotional processing. The possibility of home-based administration following appropriate training represents a potential advantage for long-term stress management, though significant safety and quality control considerations currently limit this application. Animal model evidence demonstrating that prefrontal electrical stimulation can prevent stress-induced dendritic atrophy and normalize stress hormone responses provides mechanistic support for therapeutic potential, suggesting that tDCS might counteract cellular pathology resulting from chronic stress exposure. The absence of systemic drug exposure makes tDCS potentially suitable for individuals who cannot tolerate or prefer to avoid medications, pregnant women for whom pharmacological options are limited, and those concerned about long-term medication effects.

Transcranial Magnetic Stimulation (TMS)

Introduction to Transcranial Magnetic Stimulation

Transcranial magnetic stimulation represents a non-invasive neuromodulation technique that utilizes rapidly changing magnetic fields to induce electrical currents in cortical neurons, thereby modulating neural activity in targeted brain regions. Unlike transcranial direct current stimulation which applies constant weak electrical currents, TMS employs electromagnetic induction principles where a magnetic coil positioned against the scalp generates brief, powerful magnetic pulses that pass through the skull largely unimpeded and induce secondary electrical currents in underlying cortical tissue. These induced currents can depolarize neurons and trigger action potentials when pulses exceed threshold intensity.

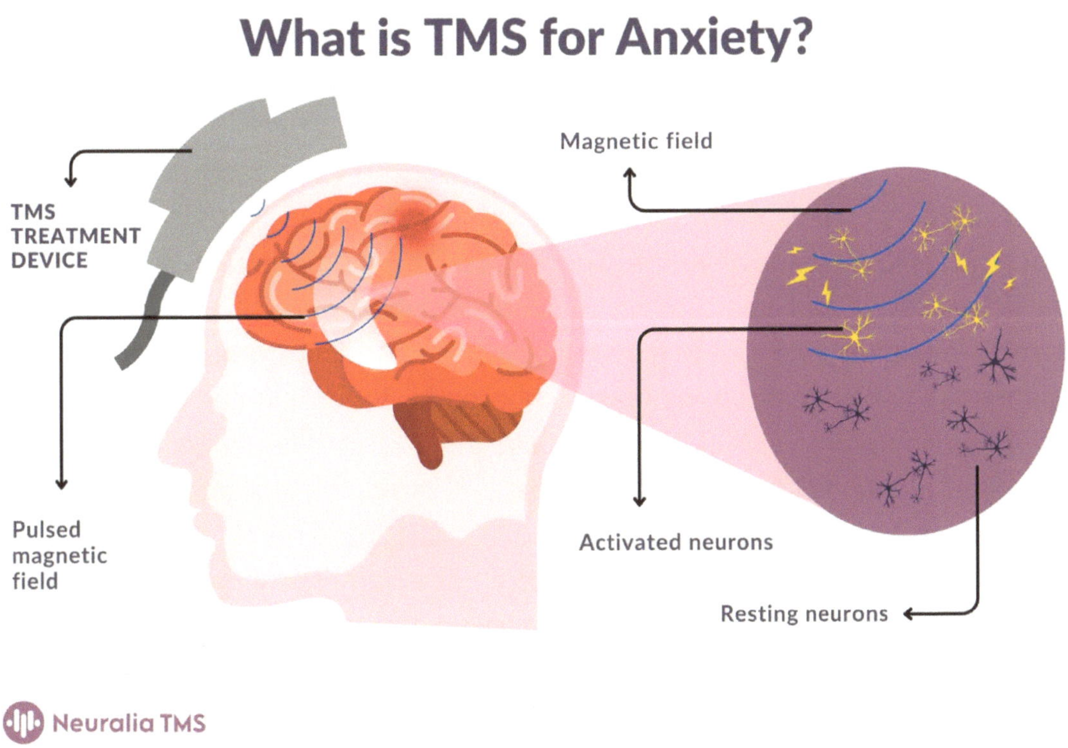

The technique exists in several forms with distinct characteristics and applications. Single-pulse TMS delivers individual magnetic pulses and is primarily used for neurophysiological assessment rather than therapeutic intervention. Paired-pulse TMS applies two pulses in rapid succession to examine cortical excitability and inhibitory mechanisms. Repetitive TMS, the form most extensively investigated for psychiatric applications, delivers trains of pulses at specific frequencies over extended periods, producing cumulative effects on cortical excitability that persist beyond the stimulation session.

The frequency of repetitive TMS critically determines its effects on cortical excitability. Low-frequency stimulation, typically defined as 1 Hz or below, generally reduces cortical excitability and neural activity in the stimulated region, producing inhibitory effects that may persist for minutes to hours following stimulation cessation. High-frequency stimulation, typically 5 Hz and above, generally increases cortical excitability and enhances neural activity, with facilitatory effects similarly outlasting the stimulation period. These frequency-dependent effects enable targeting of either hypoactive or hyperactive brain regions depending on the pathophysiology of specific conditions.

Theta burst stimulation represents a specialized TMS protocol delivering bursts of high-frequency pulses at intervals corresponding to the theta frequency range observed in hippocampal rhythms. Continuous theta burst stimulation, where bursts are delivered without interruption, produces inhibitory effects similar to low-frequency repetitive TMS but achieves comparable effects in much shorter stimulation times, typically three minutes compared to 30-40 minutes for conventional low-frequency protocols. Intermittent theta burst stimulation, where brief periods of burst stimulation alternate with rest intervals, produces facilitatory effects analogous to high-frequency repetitive TMS but similarly requires much shorter administration times. These theta burst protocols have garnered increasing interest for their efficiency and potential to enhance clinical practicality.

The mechanisms through which TMS produces therapeutic effects appear to involve multiple processes operating across different timescales. Immediate effects during stimulation include direct activation or inhibition of cortical neurons and modulation of neural network activity. Short-term aftereffects persisting minutes to hours beyond stimulation involve synaptic plasticity mechanisms including long-term potentiation and long-term depression, the cellular processes underlying learning and memory. Longer-term effects accumulating over treatment courses involving daily sessions across weeks may involve more substantial neuroplastic changes including alterations in synaptic strength, dendritic morphology, neurotrophic factor expression, and potentially structural brain changes.

Application to Chronic Stress

Transcranial magnetic stimulation offers several compelling advantages as a potential approach for managing chronic stress and stress-related symptoms. The non-invasive nature of the technique represents a fundamental advantage, as TMS requires no surgical procedures, no anesthesia, and involves no systemic drug exposure, potentially appealing to individuals seeking alternatives to pharmacological interventions or who experience intolerable medication side effects. The technique's capacity to selectively target specific cortical regions enables precise modulation of brain areas implicated in stress pathophysiology, particularly the dorsolateral prefrontal cortex which demonstrates consistent hypoactivity in chronically stressed individuals and plays critical roles in executive function, emotion regulation, and cognitive control over stress responses.

Research evidence, while preliminary, suggests several potential benefits of TMS for stress management. Studies examining healthy volunteers exposed to acute laboratory stressors have demonstrated that repetitive TMS applied to prefrontal regions may attenuate physiological stress responses including cortisol elevation, suggesting direct modulation of hypothalamic-pituitary-adrenal axis reactivity through cortical influences. These findings indicate that TMS might address a fundamental mechanism underlying chronic stress—dysregulated stress hormone responses that contribute to allostatic load and numerous adverse health consequences. The ability to normalize HPA axis function without systemic pharmacological intervention represents a significant potential advantage, as medications targeting stress responses often produce widespread effects throughout the body.

Investigations in occupationally stressed populations have provided encouraging preliminary evidence, with some studies reporting that multi-session repetitive

TMS protocols targeting left dorsolateral prefrontal cortex may reduce perceived stress levels, improve sleep quality, and enhance cognitive performance in individuals experiencing chronic work-related stress. Healthcare workers, a population experiencing particularly high occupational stress burdens, showed improvements in stress-related symptoms and better maintenance of cognitive function under demanding work conditions following TMS intervention courses in exploratory studies. These findings suggest that TMS might help individuals maintain cognitive and emotional functioning despite ongoing stressor exposure, potentially breaking the cycle where stress impairs coping capacity which further amplifies stress perception.

The demonstrated capacity of TMS to enhance prefrontal cortex function offers advantages for addressing multiple stress-related impairments simultaneously. Chronic stress typically produces a constellation of cognitive and emotional difficulties including impaired working memory, reduced attention control, difficulty making decisions, impaired emotion regulation, and tendency toward automatic negative thinking patterns. By enhancing prefrontal cortex activity and function, TMS may simultaneously address these multiple domains, potentially offering more comprehensive benefits than interventions targeting single symptoms. Research has shown that repetitive TMS can improve working memory performance, enhance attention control, and facilitate cognitive flexibility—all capacities that become compromised under chronic stress and that contribute to effective stress management when functioning optimally.

The potential for TMS to promote neuroplasticity and potentially reverse stress-induced cellular changes represents another significant advantage. Animal research has demonstrated that chronic stress produces dendritic atrophy in prefrontal cortex neurons, reduces synaptic density, and impairs synaptic plasticity mechanisms. Studies examining repetitive brain stimulation in animal stress models have shown that stimulation protocols can prevent or reverse some of these structural changes, restore synaptic plasticity, and normalize stress-responsive behaviors. If similar neuroplastic effects occur in humans receiving TMS for stress-related symptoms, the intervention might address underlying cellular pathology rather than merely providing symptomatic relief, potentially offering more durable benefits.

The objective, measurable nature of TMS represents an advantage over some psychological interventions where treatment delivery and dose are difficult to quantify precisely. Stimulation parameters including pulse frequency, intensity, number of pulses per session, and total number of sessions can be specified exactly and replicated consistently, enabling systematic investigation of dose-response relationships and optimization of protocols. This objectivity facilitates comparison across studies and eventual standardization of treatment protocols if efficacy is established. Additionally, the largely operator-independent nature of treatment delivery, once parameters are set, reduces variability introduced by therapist skill or technique differences that can influence psychological intervention outcomes.

The compatibility of TMS with concurrent psychological interventions represents another advantage. Unlike some pharmacological approaches that might interfere with cognitive-behavioral therapy processes or dull emotional experiences needed for exposure-based interventions, TMS appears compatible with and may potentially enhance psychotherapeutic approaches. The hypothesized mechanism involves TMS-induced enhancement of prefrontal neuroplasticity facilitating the learning and cognitive restructuring processes central to many psychological interventions. Preliminary research combining repetitive TMS with cognitive training suggests that stimulation may enhance training-induced improvements, supporting the possibility of synergistic effects when TMS is paired with stress management interventions teaching coping skills, relaxation techniques, or cognitive reappraisal strategies.

Research examining TMS effects on emotion regulation capabilities has demonstrated that prefrontal stimulation may enhance the capacity to implement cognitive reappraisal strategies for managing negative emotions, a skill centrally important for stress management. Studies using emotional regulation tasks have shown that individuals receiving active TMS demonstrate improved ability to reduce negative emotional responses to aversive stimuli through cognitive reappraisal compared to sham-stimulated controls. This suggests that TMS might not only directly reduce stress symptoms but also enhance the effectiveness of cognitive coping strategies, potentially providing skills that persist beyond the treatment course and help prevent future stress-related difficulties.

Application to Anxiety Disorders

Transcranial magnetic stimulation offers several potential advantages for managing anxiety disorders, with the evidence base somewhat more developed than for chronic stress though still requiring substantial additional research. The capacity to modulate prefrontal cortex activity represents a primary advantage, as anxiety disorders consistently demonstrate prefrontal hypofunction and impaired top-down regulatory control over threat-detection systems including the amygdala. By enhancing prefrontal cortex activity through high-frequency repetitive TMS or intermittent theta burst stimulation, the intervention may restore effective regulatory control, reducing excessive anxiety responses and improving capacity to implement anxiety management strategies.

Research examining repetitive TMS for generalized anxiety disorder has provided preliminary evidence of potential benefits, with several small studies reporting reductions in worry, general anxiety symptoms, and associated distress following multi-session treatment courses. Participants receiving active stimulation targeting left dorsolateral prefrontal cortex demonstrated greater symptom improvements compared to those receiving sham stimulation in controlled trials, suggesting genuine neurobiological effects beyond placebo responses. The observed reductions in worry—the central feature of generalized anxiety disorder—represent particularly meaningful outcomes, as chronic worry substantially impairs quality of life and proves difficult to control despite recognition of its excessiveness.

For panic disorder, emerging research suggests that repetitive TMS targeting prefrontal regions may reduce panic attack frequency and anticipatory anxiety between attacks. Studies examining individuals with panic disorder have reported that participants receiving active stimulation experienced fewer panic attacks during treatment courses and reduced fear of future attacks compared to baseline levels. The capacity to reduce panic frequency without systemic pharmacological intervention represents a significant advantage, as panic disorder medications often produce sedation, cognitive dulling, or carry dependence risks with benzodiazepines. Additionally, some preliminary evidence suggests that TMS may reduce interoceptive sensitivity—the excessive awareness of bodily sensations that characterizes panic disorder—potentially addressing a maintaining factor in the condition.

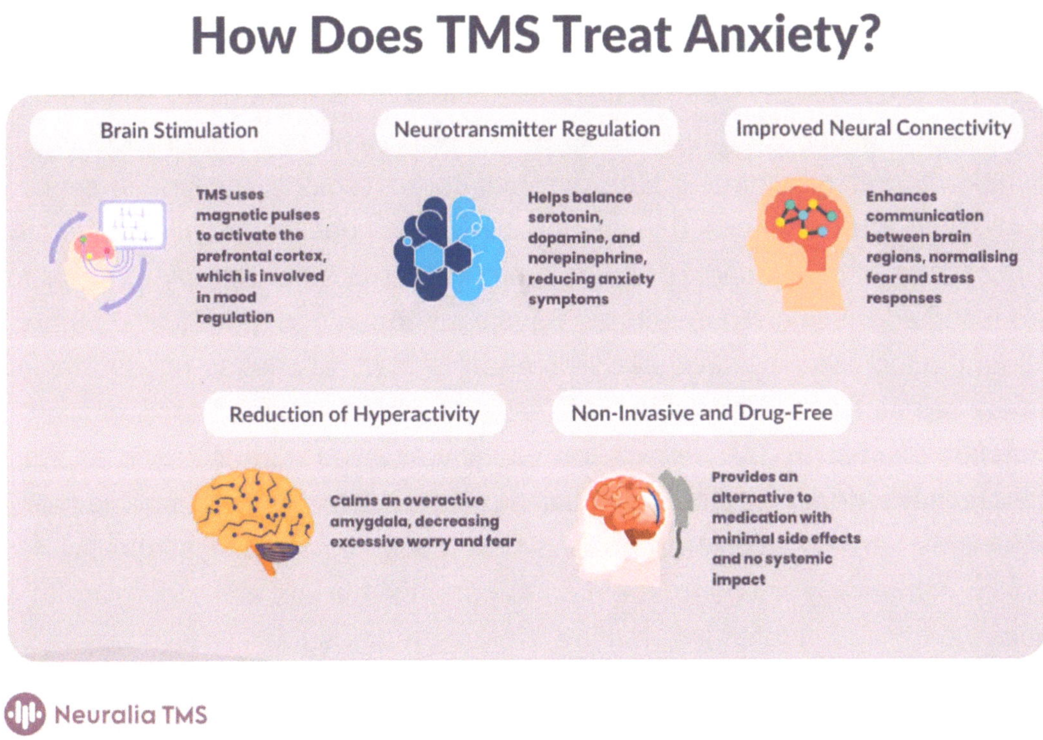

Research investigating TMS for social anxiety disorder has explored whether enhancing prefrontal function might reduce fear of social evaluation and improve social functioning. Studies have demonstrated that individuals with social anxiety receiving repetitive TMS targeting left dorsolateral prefrontal cortex show reductions in social anxiety symptoms, decreased fear responses to social threat cues such as negative facial expressions, and improvements in performance during social interaction tasks. The capacity to reduce amygdala hyperreactivity to social threats through prefrontal stimulation represents a mechanistic advantage, as neuroimaging studies have demonstrated that TMS can modulate functional connectivity between prefrontal cortex and amygdala, potentially enhancing top-down inhibitory control.

The potential for TMS to facilitate extinction learning represents a particularly important advantage for anxiety disorders, where impaired extinction—difficulty learning that previously feared situations are now safe—represents a core maintaining mechanism. Preclinical research in animal models has demonstrated that repetitive brain stimulation targeting prefrontal regions can enhance extinction of conditioned fear responses, and preliminary human studies suggest similar effects. For post-traumatic stress disorder, research has examined whether TMS can facilitate extinction of trauma-related fear, with some evidence suggesting that stimulation targeting ventromedial prefrontal cortex regions involved in extinction consolidation may enhance the effectiveness of exposure-based interventions. The possibility of combining TMS with prolonged exposure therapy or other trauma-focused approaches represents a significant advantage, potentially enhancing treatment outcomes for individuals who show limited responses to psychological interventions alone.

Studies examining TMS effects on cognitive biases characteristic of anxiety disorders have demonstrated potential advantages for addressing maintaining mechanisms. Anxiety involves attentional bias toward threatening stimuli, with individuals automatically orienting attention to potential threats and struggling to disengage from threat-related information. Research has shown that repetitive TMS targeting dorsolateral prefrontal cortex may reduce attentional bias toward threat, enabling more balanced attention allocation and reducing the hypervigilance that maintains anxiety. Similarly, interpretation bias—the tendency to interpret ambiguous situations as threatening—may be modifiable through TMS-enhanced cognitive control, though research remains preliminary.

The capacity of TMS to modulate physiological arousal represents another potential advantage for anxiety management. Anxiety disorders involve chronic autonomic hyperarousal with elevated heart rate, increased blood pressure, muscle tension, and other physiological manifestations. Research examining repetitive TMS effects on autonomic function has suggested that prefrontal stimulation may reduce sympathetic nervous system activity and enhance parasympathetic tone, potentially normalizing the autonomic imbalance characteristic of anxiety. Some studies have reported reductions in resting heart rate, decreased heart rate variability abnormalities, and reduced physiological reactivity to stressors following TMS treatment courses, suggesting effects on brainstem autonomic control centers potentially mediated through prefrontal-brainstem connections.

For individuals with anxiety disorders who have not responded adequately to first-line interventions including cognitive-behavioral therapy and medication approaches, TMS represents a potential alternative that addresses neural circuit dysfunction through a different mechanism. The availability of additional intervention options for treatment-resistant anxiety may prevent progression to more severe disability and improve long-term outcomes. Research specifically examining TMS in treatment-resistant anxiety populations remains limited but preliminary findings suggest that some individuals who have not benefited from multiple prior interventions may show responses to TMS protocols, indicating the technique addresses aspects of pathophysiology not adequately targeted by conventional approaches.

Application to Major Depressive Disorder

Transcranial magnetic stimulation for major depressive disorder represents the most extensively researched and clinically advanced psychiatric application of the technique, with substantially more robust evidence supporting efficacy compared to applications for stress or anxiety. The intervention received regulatory approval from the United States Food and Drug Administration in 2008 for treatment-resistant depression, representing formal recognition of its therapeutic potential and establishing TMS as a legitimate intervention option within the psychiatric treatment armamentarium. This regulatory approval provides confidence regarding safety and efficacy that remains absent for most other neuromodulation approaches to psychiatric conditions.

The advantages of TMS for depression begin with addressing a critical unmet clinical need—treatment-resistant depression affects approximately one-third of individuals with major depressive disorder who do not achieve remission despite adequate trials of multiple antidepressant medications. For these individuals, options become increasingly limited, often involving medication combinations, augmentation strategies, or electroconvulsive therapy. TMS offers an alternative with a distinct mechanism of action that may benefit individuals whose depression has not responded to pharmacological approaches, potentially because TMS addresses circuit-level dysfunction not adequately modulated by systemic drug interventions targeting specific neurotransmitter systems.

Extensive research evidence supports TMS efficacy for depression, with multiple large-scale randomized controlled trials, systematic reviews, and meta-analyses consistently demonstrating that active repetitive TMS produces superior antidepressant effects compared to sham stimulation. Effect sizes, while variable across studies, generally fall in the medium range and appear comparable to those observed for antidepressant medications in head-to-head comparison studies. Some research suggests that TMS may produce response rates of 50-60% and remission rates of 30-40% in treatment-resistant populations, representing meaningful clinical benefit for individuals who have exhausted multiple medication options. The consistency of positive findings across numerous independent investigations conducted in different countries with diverse populations provides strong evidence for genuine therapeutic effects.

The favorable safety profile of TMS compared to some alternative interventions for severe or treatment-resistant depression represents a significant advantage. Electroconvulsive therapy, while highly effective, requires general anesthesia, intentionally induces seizures, and frequently produces cognitive side effects, including memory impairment, that some individuals find unacceptable. TMS requires no anesthesia, does not induce seizures when administered according to established safety parameters, and cognitive assessments have generally not revealed significant adverse cognitive effects, with some studies suggest possible cognitive improvements. This safety advantage may encourage earlier consideration of TMS in treatment algorithms rather than reserving it only for individuals who have failed numerous other approaches.

Research has demonstrated that TMS produces measurable changes in brain function and connectivity that correlate with clinical improvement, providing evidence that therapeutic effects reflect genuine neurobiological mechanisms rather than placebo responses. Neuroimaging studies have shown that successful TMS treatment normalizes prefrontal cortex hypoactivity characteristic of depression, enhances functional connectivity between prefrontal regulatory regions and limbic emotional regions, and modulates default mode network hyperactivity associated with rumination. Positron emission tomography research has demonstrated that TMS influences neurotransmitter systems including serotonin and dopamine, potentially explaining mechanisms through which focal cortical stimulation produces distributed effects on mood-regulating networks.

The capacity of TMS to address specific symptom dimensions of depression represents an advantage for personalized intervention approaches. Research examining which depressive symptoms respond most robustly to TMS has suggested that cognitive symptoms including concentration difficulties, indecisiveness, and mental slowing may show particularly good responses, potentially reflecting direct enhancement of dorsolateral prefrontal cortex function. Some evidence suggests that anhedonia—the inability to experience pleasure—may improve with TMS, possibly through modulation of reward circuitry via prefrontal-striatal connections. The possibility of matching intervention approaches to individual symptom profiles could enable more targeted, effective treatment strategies.

For individuals who cannot tolerate antidepressant medications due to side effects, medical contraindications, or personal preference, TMS provides an option that avoids systemic drug exposure and associated adverse effects including weight gain, sexual dysfunction, gastrointestinal disturbances, or metabolic changes. Pregnant women, for whom most antidepressant medications carry some degree of fetal risk or inadequate safety data, may find TMS an appealing option, though research specifically examining TMS during pregnancy remains extremely limited and considerable caution is warranted. Elderly individuals who often experience medication side effects more severely and metabolize drugs differently may benefit from TMS as an alternative that avoids pharmacokinetic complications, though age-related brain changes may influence treatment response.

The demonstrated capacity of TMS to promote neuroplasticity and potentially reverse cellular pathology in depression represents a mechanistic advantage. Research has suggested that repetitive TMS increases brain-derived neurotrophic factor expression, enhances synaptic plasticity, promotes synaptogenesis, and may even stimulate neurogenesis in hippocampus based on animal studies. If TMS induces similar neuroplastic changes in humans, the intervention may address the synaptic deficits, dendritic atrophy, and impaired plasticity that characterize depression at the cellular level, potentially providing more fundamental therapeutic effects than medications that primarily modulate neurotransmitter levels without directly promoting structural brain changes.

Research examining long-term outcomes following TMS for depression has provided evidence that some individuals maintain improvements for extended periods, with some studies reporting sustained remission months to years after acute treatment courses. The possibility of achieving durable benefits without requiring continuous intervention represents a significant advantage compared to antidepressant medications which typically require indefinite continuation to prevent relapse. While many individuals do eventually experience symptom recurrence, retreatment with TMS appears feasible and may re-establish therapeutic benefits, and maintenance protocols involving periodic sessions have shown promise for sustaining improvements in preliminary studies.

Hyperbaric Oxygenation Therapy with Hyperbaric Oxygen Chamber (HBOT)

Introduction to Hyperbaric Oxygen Therapy

Hyperbaric oxygen therapy represents a medical intervention involving the administration of pure oxygen or oxygen-enriched air at pressures exceeding normal atmospheric pressure, typically delivered within a specialized chamber designed to withstand elevated pressures. The fundamental principle underlying hyperbaric oxygen therapy involves increasing the amount of oxygen dissolved in blood plasma and body tissues beyond levels achievable through normal breathing at sea-level atmospheric pressure. Standard atmospheric pressure at sea level measures approximately 1 atmosphere absolute, while therapeutic hyperbaric protocols typically employ pressures ranging from 1.5 to 3.0 atmospheres absolute, with most psychiatric applications utilizing pressures in the lower to middle portion of this range.

The physics governing hyperbaric oxygen therapy derive from gas laws, particularly Henry's law, which states that the amount of gas dissolved in a liquid is directly proportional to the partial pressure of that gas above the liquid. By increasing ambient pressure and delivering concentrated oxygen, hyperbaric conditions dramatically increase the partial pressure of oxygen, resulting in substantially elevated dissolved oxygen concentrations in blood plasma. Under normal conditions at sea level breathing room air, approximately 98% of oxygen transport occurs bound to hemoglobin in red blood cells, with only about 2% dissolved in plasma. Under hyperbaric conditions breathing pure oxygen, dissolved oxygen in plasma can increase fifteen-fold or more, providing oxygen delivery independent of hemoglobin and reaching tissues with compromised blood flow.

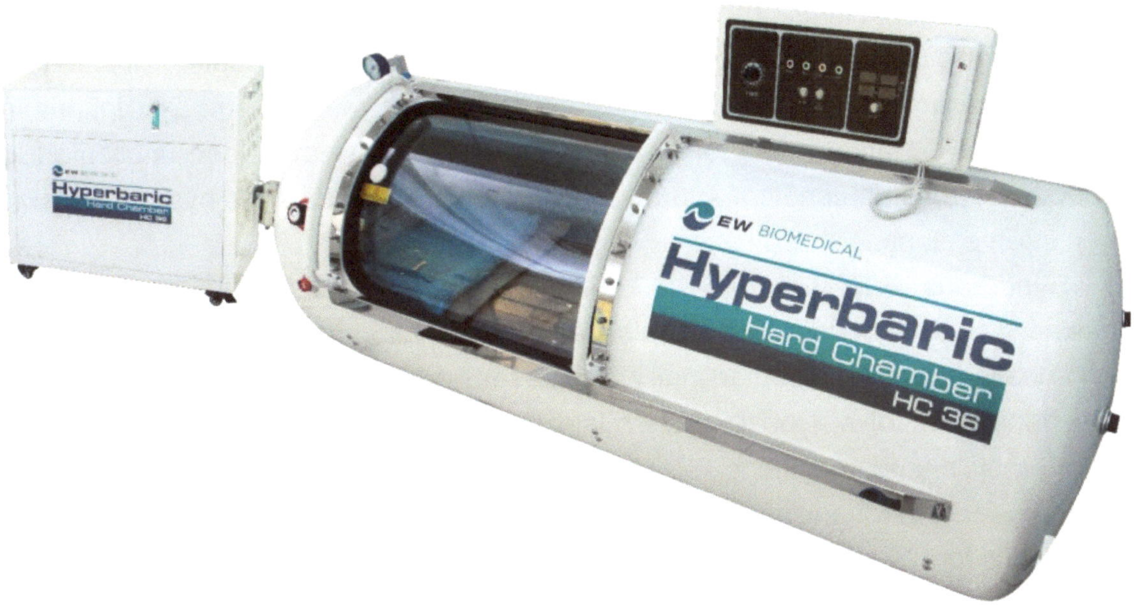

Source: European Wellness

Hyperbaric oxygen therapy protocols vary in pressure, oxygen concentration, session duration, and treatment course length. Typical sessions last 60 to 120 minutes, during which patients breathe pure oxygen or oxygen-enriched air through a mask or hood, or simply breathe the pressurized chamber atmosphere if the entire chamber is filled with oxygen. Monoplace chambers accommodate single patients and are typically pressurized entirely with oxygen, while multiplace chambers hold multiple patients and staff, with patients breathing oxygen through masks while the chamber itself is pressurized with compressed air. Treatment courses for chronic conditions typically involve daily or near-daily sessions over several weeks, with total courses ranging from 20 to 60 sessions, depending on the condition and protocol employed.

The proposed mechanisms through which hyperbaric oxygen therapy might influence brain function and psychiatric symptoms are multifaceted and incompletely understood. Hyperoxia, the state of elevated tissue oxygen levels, may influence cellular metabolism, mitochondrial function, oxidative stress pathways, inflammatory processes, neurotransmitter systems, vascular function, and neuroplasticity mechanisms. The brain, despite comprising only approximately 2% of body weight, consumes roughly 20% of the body's oxygen supply, reflecting its high metabolic demands and dependence on aerobic metabolism. Disruptions in cerebral oxygenation, metabolism, or vascular function have been implicated in various psychiatric conditions, providing theoretical rationale for hyperbaric oxygen interventions.

Hyperbaric oxygen therapy has established efficacy for various medical conditions including decompression sickness, carbon monoxide poisoning, chronic non-healing wounds, radiation injury, and several other approved indications where mechanisms involve hypoxia, ischemia, or impaired wound healing. The application to psychiatric conditions represents a more speculative extension based on hypothesized mechanisms involving cerebral metabolism, inflammation, or vascular function, with considerably less robust evidence compared to established medical indications.

Application to Chronic Stress

Hyperbaric oxygen therapy offers several potential advantages for managing chronic stress, though research specifically examining this application remains extremely limited and largely confined to animal models and small exploratory human studies. The capacity to enhance cerebral oxygen delivery represents a fundamental advantage, as chronic stress has been associated with alterations in cerebral blood flow and metabolism that might be addressed through hyperoxia. Neuroimaging studies of chronically stressed individuals have revealed reduced cerebral blood flow in prefrontal regions and other areas involved in stress regulation, suggesting potential vascular contributions to stress-related symptoms that could theoretically benefit from enhanced oxygen delivery.

Animal research examining chronic stress models has provided preliminary evidence suggesting potential benefits of hyperbaric oxygen interventions. Studies subjecting rodents to chronic unpredictable stress or repeated restraint stress have demonstrated that hyperbaric oxygen sessions can reduce behavioral indicators of stress, normalize stress hormone responses, and prevent some neurobiological changes associated with chronic stress exposure. These animal studies have shown that hyperbaric oxygen may attenuate stress-induced elevation in corticosterone levels, reduce anxiety-like behaviors in stress-exposed animals, and preserve hippocampal neurogenesis that chronic stress typically suppresses. While translating findings from animal models to human applications requires substantial caution, these studies provide mechanistic support for potential therapeutic effects.

The proposed anti-inflammatory effects of hyperbaric oxygen therapy represent another potential advantage for stress management, as chronic stress is associated with elevated inflammatory markers and neuroinflammation that contribute to stress-related pathology. Research has suggested that hyperbaric oxygen may modulate inflammatory processes through multiple mechanisms, including effects on immune cell function, cytokine production, and inflammatory signaling pathways. Some studies have reported that hyperbaric oxygen can reduce pro-inflammatory cytokine levels, including interleukin-6 and tumor necrosis factor-alpha, while enhancing anti-inflammatory mediators, creating a profile that might counteract stress-induced inflammatory activation. The possibility of reducing neuroinflammation without systemic immunosuppressive medications represents a significant theoretical advantage.

Hyperbaric oxygen therapy's potential effects on mitochondrial function offer another avenue through which the intervention might address stress-related symptoms. Chronic stress has been associated with mitochondrial dysfunction, oxidative stress, and impaired cellular energy metabolism that contribute to fatigue, cognitive dysfunction, and other symptoms accompanying chronic stress. Hyperbaric oxygen has been proposed to enhance mitochondrial function through multiple mechanisms, including increased oxidative phosphorylation efficiency, stimulation of mitochondrial biogenesis, and modulation of oxidative stress pathways. Some research has suggested that intermittent hyperoxia may trigger adaptive responses that enhance cellular stress resistance and improve energy metabolism, potentially addressing the metabolic dysfunction associated with chronic stress.

Small exploratory studies examining hyperbaric oxygen in stressed populations have reported preliminary findings suggesting potential benefits. Research investigating individuals with stress-related exhaustion syndrome, a condition recognized in some classification systems involving severe fatigue and cognitive dysfunction following prolonged stress, has reported improvements in fatigue, cognitive performance, and quality of life following hyperbaric oxygen treatment courses. While these studies typically lack rigorous control groups and involve small samples, the consistency of reported improvements across multiple domains suggests possible genuine effects worthy of more systematic investigation.

The capacity of hyperbaric oxygen to potentially enhance neuroplasticity represents another theoretical advantage for stress management. Research has suggested that hyperbaric conditions may promote expression of neurotrophic factors, including brain-derived neurotrophic factor and vascular endothelial growth factor, molecules that support neuronal survival, synaptic plasticity, and angiogenesis. Chronic stress reduces BDNF expression and impairs neuroplasticity, contributing to structural brain changes including hippocampal atrophy and prefrontal dendritic retraction. If hyperbaric oxygen enhances neurotrophic support, the intervention might counteract stress-induced cellular pathology and promote recovery of brain structure and function.

Application to Anxiety Disorders

Hyperbaric oxygen therapy presents several potential advantages for anxiety disorder management, though research specifically examining this application remains nascent, with evidence derived primarily from case reports, small case series, and exploratory studies lacking rigorous controls. The intervention's capacity to modulate brain metabolism and function through enhanced oxygen delivery provides a mechanistic rationale for its potential anxiolytic effects, as anxiety disorders involve alterations in neural activity patterns, neurotransmitter function, and metabolic activity in brain regions such as the prefrontal cortex, amygdala, and insula.

Case reports and small series examining individuals with various anxiety disorders who received hyperbaric oxygen therapy have described reductions in anxiety symptoms, decreased panic attack frequency, improved stress tolerance, and enhanced overall functioning. While the uncontrolled nature of these reports' limits interpretability and publication bias likely favors positive outcomes, the consistency of reported improvements across multiple case descriptions suggests possible genuine effects. Some individuals with treatment-resistant anxiety who had shown limited responses to multiple conventional interventions reportedly experienced meaningful symptom reductions following hyperbaric oxygen treatment courses, suggesting the intervention may address aspects of pathophysiology not adequately targeted by standard approaches.

The proposed effects of hyperbaric oxygen on gamma-aminobutyric acid neurotransmission represent a potential mechanism through which the intervention might produce anxiolytic effects. GABA, the primary inhibitory neurotransmitter in the brain, plays critical roles in regulating anxiety, with reduced GABAergic function implicated in anxiety disorder pathophysiology. Some research has suggested that hyperbaric oxygen may influence GABAergic neurotransmission, potentially enhancing inhibitory tone and reducing neural hyperexcitability characteristic of anxiety states. While mechanisms remain speculative, the possibility of enhancing GABAergic function without pharmacological interventions that carry dependence risks represents a theoretical advantage.

Research examining hyperbaric oxygen effects on autonomic nervous system function has suggested that the intervention may promote parasympathetic activation and reduce sympathetic hyperactivity, potentially normalizing the autonomic imbalance characteristic of anxiety disorders. Studies measuring heart rate variability, a marker of autonomic function, have reported increases in parasympathetic indices following hyperbaric oxygen sessions, suggesting enhanced vagal tone associated with relaxation and reduced anxiety. The capacity to directly modulate autonomic function through a physical intervention represents an advantage for addressing the physiological manifestations of anxiety, including rapid heart rate, elevated blood pressure, and chronic muscle tension.

Animal studies examining anxiety-like behaviors have provided some mechanistic support for potential anxiolytic effects of hyperbaric oxygen. Research using established animal models of anxiety has demonstrated that hyperbaric oxygen sessions can reduce anxiety-like behaviors in tests such as the elevated plus maze and open field paradigms. These studies have shown that hyperbaric-treated animals spend more time in anxiety-provoking areas, demonstrate reduced freezing behavior, and show normalization of stress hormone responses compared to control animals. While animal anxiety models imperfectly represent human anxiety disorders, these findings suggest neurobiological effects relevant to anxiety regulation.

The potential for hyperbaric oxygen to enhance cerebral blood flow and correct regional perfusion abnormalities represents another advantage for anxiety management. Some neuroimaging research has suggested that anxiety disorders may involve altered cerebral blood flow patterns, with some regions showing hypoperfusion and others demonstrating increased perfusion. Hyperbaric oxygen's capacity to enhance oxygen delivery to relatively hypoxic regions while potentially normalizing vascular function could theoretically address these perfusion abnormalities. The absence of systemic pharmacological effects makes this approach potentially suitable for individuals who cannot tolerate anxiolytic medications or prefer non-pharmacological interventions.

Application to Major Depressive Disorder

Hyperbaric oxygen therapy offers several potential advantages for major depressive disorder management, with more substantial research evidence compared to applications for stress or anxiety, though the evidence base remains considerably less developed than for established depression interventions. The capacity to enhance cerebral metabolism and oxygen delivery provides theoretical rationale for antidepressant effects, as depression has been associated with reduced cerebral blood flow, decreased glucose metabolism, and alterations in oxidative metabolism in the prefrontal cortex, anterior cingulate cortex, and other mood-regulating regions identified through neuroimaging studies.

Multiple small clinical trials examining hyperbaric oxygen therapy for depression have reported encouraging findings, with several studies demonstrating significant reductions in depressive symptom severity following treatment courses. Research involving individuals with treatment-resistant depression who had not responded adequately to multiple antidepressant medications has shown that substantial proportions of participants experienced clinically meaningful improvements following hyperbaric oxygen protocols, with some studies reporting response rates of 40-60%. These findings suggest that hyperbaric oxygen may benefit some individuals whose depression has proven refractory to conventional pharmacological approaches, potentially because the intervention addresses pathophysiological mechanisms not adequately modulated by medications targeting monoamine neurotransmitters.

The proposed anti-inflammatory effects of hyperbaric oxygen represent a particularly relevant advantage for depression, given the growing recognition of inflammation's role in depressive pathophysiology. Research has demonstrated that approximately 30-40% of depressed individuals show elevated inflammatory markers, including C-reactive protein, interleukin-6, and tumor necrosis factor-alpha, and this inflammatory subtype often shows reduced responses to conventional antidepressants. Studies examining hyperbaric oxygen effects on inflammatory markers have reported reductions in pro-inflammatory cytokines and increases in anti-inflammatory mediators, suggesting potential specific benefits for inflammatory depression. The capacity to address inflammation through a physical intervention, avoiding systemic immunosuppression, represents a significant theoretical advantage for this depression subtype.

Research examining hyperbaric oxygen effects on brain-derived neurotrophic factor has provided mechanistic support for potential antidepressant effects, as BDNF plays critical roles in neuroplasticity, neurogenesis, and resilience to stress, with depression characterized by reduced BDNF expression. Animal studies have demonstrated that hyperbaric oxygen can increase hippocampal BDNF levels, enhance neurogenesis in the dentate gyrus, and promote synaptic plasticity. Some human research has reported increases in serum BDNF levels following hyperbaric oxygen treatment courses, though whether peripheral BDNF levels reflect brain concentrations remains uncertain. If hyperbaric oxygen enhances neurotrophic support in the brain, the intervention might address cellular pathology underlying depression, including synaptic deficits, dendritic atrophy, and impaired neuroplasticity.

The potential for hyperbaric oxygen to improve mitochondrial function and cellular energy metabolism offers another mechanism through which the intervention might produce antidepressant effects. Depression has been associated with mitochondrial dysfunction, reduced ATP production, and impaired oxidative phosphorylation in brain, contributing to symptoms including fatigue, cognitive dysfunction, and reduced motivation. Studies examining hyperbaric oxygen effects on mitochondrial function have suggested that the intervention may enhance mitochondrial respiratory capacity, promote mitochondrial biogenesis, and improve cellular energy status. The possibility of addressing metabolic dysfunction contributing to depression represents an advantage for symptoms, including fatigue and anhedonia, that often respond poorly to conventional antidepressants.

Neuroimaging research examining hyperbaric oxygen effects in depression has demonstrated changes in brain function and metabolism that may correlate with clinical improvement. Studies using single-photon emission computed tomography or positron emission tomography have reported that hyperbaric oxygen treatment courses can increase cerebral blood flow and metabolism in hypofunctioning prefrontal and anterior cingulate regions, potentially normalizing the hypometabolism characteristic of depression. Functional MRI studies have suggested that hyperbaric oxygen may modulate activity in mood-regulating networks, including default mode and salience networks, with changes in network function correlating with symptom improvements.

For individuals with depression who cannot tolerate or prefer to avoid antidepressant medications, hyperbaric oxygen provides an alternative approach that involves no systemic drug exposure, avoiding medication side effects, including weight gain, sexual dysfunction, or metabolic disturbances. The intervention may be particularly appealing for individuals with medical conditions complicating pharmacological management, those experiencing intolerable medication side effects, or individuals philosophically opposed to psychotropic medication use. The capacity to achieve antidepressant effects through a physical intervention targeting brain metabolism and function represents a conceptually distinct approach from neurotransmitter-focused pharmacotherapy.

Ozone Therapy

Introduction to Ozone Therapy

Ozone therapy represents a complementary medical approach involving the therapeutic application of ozone, a molecule composed of three oxygen atoms (O_3) rather than the two atoms found in standard molecular oxygen (O_3). The technique has been utilized in various medical contexts for over a century, with applications ranging from wound healing and infection management to more recent explorations in chronic disease management and, increasingly, psychiatric conditions. Ozone exists as a highly reactive and unstable gas that rapidly decomposes into molecular oxygen, and this reactivity underlies both its potential therapeutic mechanisms and the controversies surrounding its clinical application.

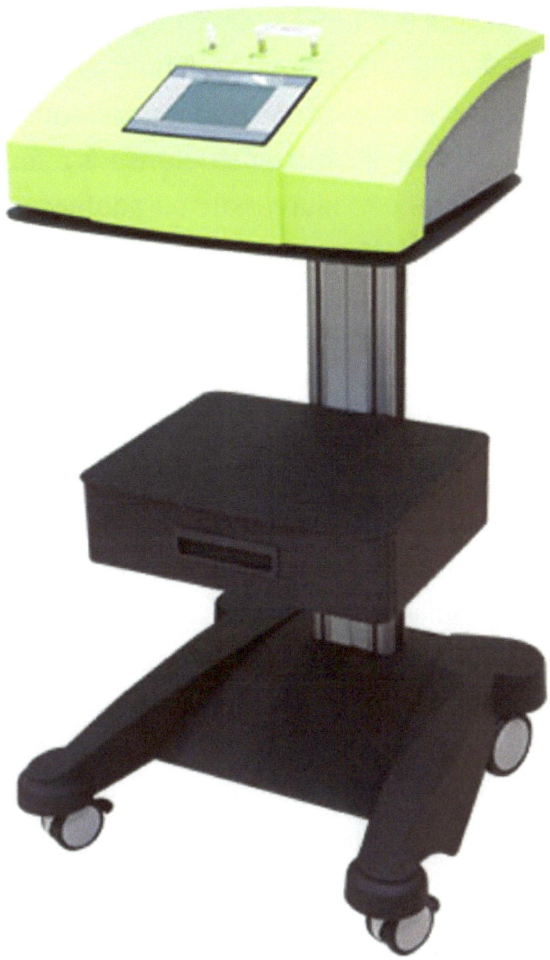

Source: European Wellness.

The administration routes for ozone therapy are diverse, reflecting the molecule's reactivity and inability to be directly inhaled into the lungs due to toxicity to the respiratory epithelium. Common methods include major autohemotherapy, where a quantity of patient blood is withdrawn, mixed with medical-grade ozone, and reinfused intravenously; minor autohemotherapy involving smaller blood volumes typically injected intramuscularly; rectal insufflation where ozone gas is introduced into the rectum; ozonated water or oil for topical or internal use; and direct intravenous injection of ozone-oxygen mixtures, though this method remains controversial and is not widely practiced due to safety concerns.

The proposed mechanisms through which ozone therapy might influence physiological function and potentially impact psychiatric symptoms involve multiple pathways. Ozone's strong oxidative properties trigger controlled oxidative stress that may paradoxically activate antioxidant defense systems through hormetic mechanisms, where mild stress exposure induces adaptive responses enhancing stress resistance. This mild oxidative challenge may stimulate expression of antioxidant enzymes including superoxide dismutase, catalase, and glutathione peroxidase, potentially improving the organism's capacity to manage oxidative stress more broadly.

Ozone therapy has been proposed to modulate immune function through effects on cytokine production, with some research suggesting that controlled ozone exposure can reduce pro-inflammatory cytokines while enhancing anti-inflammatory mediators. The technique may influence mitochondrial function and cellular metabolism, potentially enhancing oxidative phosphorylation efficiency and ATP production. Effects on blood rheology, including potential improvements in red blood cell deformability and oxygen release to tissues, have been hypothesized to enhance tissue oxygenation. Additionally, ozone may influence nitric oxide metabolism and vascular endothelial function, with potential implications for cerebral blood flow and neural function.

The application of ozone therapy to psychiatric conditions represents a relatively recent and highly exploratory area with limited rigorous research evidence. Most available literature consists of case reports, small case series, and studies conducted primarily in countries where ozone therapy enjoys greater acceptance within medical practice, particularly in parts of Europe, Latin America, and Russia.

The theoretical rationale for psychiatric applications centers on hypothesized effects on neuroinflammation, oxidative stress, mitochondrial function, and cerebral metabolism—pathophysiological processes implicated in mood and anxiety disorders.

Application to Chronic Stress

Ozone therapy presents several potential advantages for chronic stress management based on preliminary research and proposed mechanisms, though evidence remains largely confined to animal models and small exploratory human studies. The intervention's capacity to modulate oxidative stress pathways offers theoretical benefits for stress-related conditions, as chronic stress is associated with elevated oxidative stress, increased reactive oxygen species production, and depletion of antioxidant defenses. Research has suggested that controlled ozone exposure may paradoxically enhance antioxidant capacity through hormetic mechanisms, where mild oxidative stress triggers adaptive upregulation of antioxidant enzyme systems. This enhanced antioxidant capacity might counteract the oxidative damage associated with chronic stress, potentially protecting neurons and other cells from stress-induced injury.

Animal research examining stress models has provided some evidence supporting potential benefits of ozone therapy. Studies subjecting rodents to chronic stress paradigms have demonstrated that ozone administration can reduce behavioral indicators of stress, normalize stress hormone levels, and attenuate stress-induced biochemical changes. These animal studies have shown that ozone-treated stressed animals exhibit reduced anxiety-like behaviors, lower corticosterone elevation in response to stressors, and preservation of hippocampal antioxidant enzyme activities that chronic stress typically depletes. While extrapolating from animal studies to human applications requires caution, these findings suggest biological plausibility for stress-protective effects.

The proposed anti-inflammatory effects of ozone therapy represent another potential advantage for stress management, as chronic stress involves inflammatory activation that contributes to numerous stress-related health consequences. Research has suggested that ozone therapy may reduce pro-inflammatory cytokine levels, including interleukin-6, interleukin-1 beta, and tumor necrosis factor-alpha, while promoting anti-inflammatory mediators such as interleukin-10. This immunomodulatory profile could theoretically address the chronic low-grade inflammation characteristic of chronic stress without the systemic immunosuppression associated with some pharmaceutical anti-inflammatory approaches. Small human studies examining individuals with chronic stress-related conditions have reported reductions in inflammatory markers following ozone therapy courses, though these findings require replication in controlled trials.

The potential for ozone therapy to enhance mitochondrial function and cellular energy metabolism offers another theoretical advantage for stress management. Chronic stress impairs mitochondrial function, reduces ATP production, and disrupts cellular energy homeostasis, contributing to fatigue, cognitive dysfunction, and reduced stress tolerance. Ozone therapy has been proposed to stimulate mitochondrial activity through mild oxidative stress that triggers adaptive mitochondrial biogenesis and enhances oxidative phosphorylation efficiency. Some research has reported increased ATP production and improved mitochondrial respiratory capacity following ozone exposure, suggesting potential for addressing metabolic dysfunction associated with chronic stress.

Application to Anxiety Disorders

Ozone therapy offers several potential advantages for anxiety disorder management, though research specifically examining this application remains extremely limited with evidence derived primarily from case reports and small exploratory studies. The proposed anxiolytic mechanisms involve modulation of oxidative stress, inflammation, and neurotransmitter systems, providing theoretical rationale for potential benefits. Case reports describing individuals with various anxiety disorders who received ozone therapy have documented reductions in anxiety symptoms, decreased panic attack frequency, improved stress tolerance, and enhanced quality of life. While the uncontrolled nature of case reports severely limits interpretability and publication bias likely favors positive outcomes, the consistency of reported improvements across multiple descriptions suggests possible genuine effects warranting systematic investigation.

The capacity of ozone therapy to potentially modulate GABAergic neurotransmission represents a theoretical mechanism through which the intervention might produce anxiolytic effects. GABA, the primary inhibitory neurotransmitter, plays critical roles in anxiety regulation, with reduced GABAergic function implicated in anxiety pathophysiology. Some research has suggested that ozone therapy may influence brain neurotransmitter systems, potentially enhancing GABAergic activity and reducing neural hyperexcitability. Animal studies have demonstrated that ozone administration can increase brain GABA levels and enhance GABAergic receptor function, providing mechanistic support for possible anxiolytic effects. The possibility of modulating inhibitory neurotransmission without pharmacological agents that carry dependence risks represents a theoretical advantage.

Ozone therapy's proposed effects on cerebral blood flow and oxygen delivery offer another potential advantage for anxiety management. Some research has suggested that ozone therapy may improve blood rheological properties, enhance red blood cell deformability, and increase oxygen release to tissues, potentially improving cerebral oxygenation. Anxiety disorders have been associated with altered cerebral blood flow patterns, and interventions enhancing oxygen delivery to brain regions involved in anxiety regulation might theoretically produce therapeutic benefits. Small studies examining cerebral blood flow before and after ozone therapy courses have reported increased perfusion in some brain regions, though whether these changes relate to clinical improvements remains unclear.

Application to Major Depressive Disorder

Ozone therapy presents several potential advantages for major depressive disorder management, with slightly more substantial research compared to stress or anxiety applications, though evidence remains far less developed than for conventional depression interventions. The capacity to modulate multiple pathophysiological mechanisms implicated in depression including oxidative stress, inflammation, mitochondrial dysfunction, and neurotransmitter systems provides theoretical rationale for antidepressant effects. Several small clinical studies examining ozone therapy for depression have reported encouraging findings, with research demonstrating significant reductions in depressive symptom severity following treatment courses. Studies involving individuals with treatment-resistant depression have shown that meaningful proportions of participants experienced improvements following ozone therapy protocols, suggesting potential benefits for individuals whose depression has not responded adequately to conventional pharmacological approaches.

The proposed anti-inflammatory effects of ozone therapy represent a particularly relevant advantage for depression, especially for the inflammatory subtype characterized by elevated inflammatory markers. Research examining ozone therapy effects on inflammatory mediators has demonstrated reductions in pro-inflammatory cytokines and increases in anti-inflammatory markers, suggesting potential specific benefits for inflammatory depression. Studies have reported decreases in C-reactive protein, interleukin-6, and tumor necrosis factor-alpha levels following ozone therapy courses in depressed individuals, with cytokine reductions correlating with symptom improvements. The capacity to address inflammation through a biological intervention, avoiding systemic medications, represents a theoretical advantage for depression with prominent inflammatory components.

The potential for ozone therapy to enhance mitochondrial function and cellular energy metabolism offers a mechanism through which the intervention might produce antidepressant effects. Depression has been associated with mitochondrial dysfunction, impaired ATP production, and reduced oxidative phosphorylation, contributing to symptoms including fatigue, cognitive impairment, and anhedonia. Research has suggested that ozone therapy may stimulate mitochondrial biogenesis, enhance respiratory chain complex activities, and improve cellular energy status. Studies examining energy metabolism markers have reported increases in ATP levels and improvements in mitochondrial function following ozone therapy, potentially addressing metabolic dysfunction underlying depression. The possibility of improving cellular energy metabolism represents an advantage for depressive symptoms that often respond poorly to conventional antidepressants, particularly fatigue and reduced motivation.

Bio Hormonal Modulator

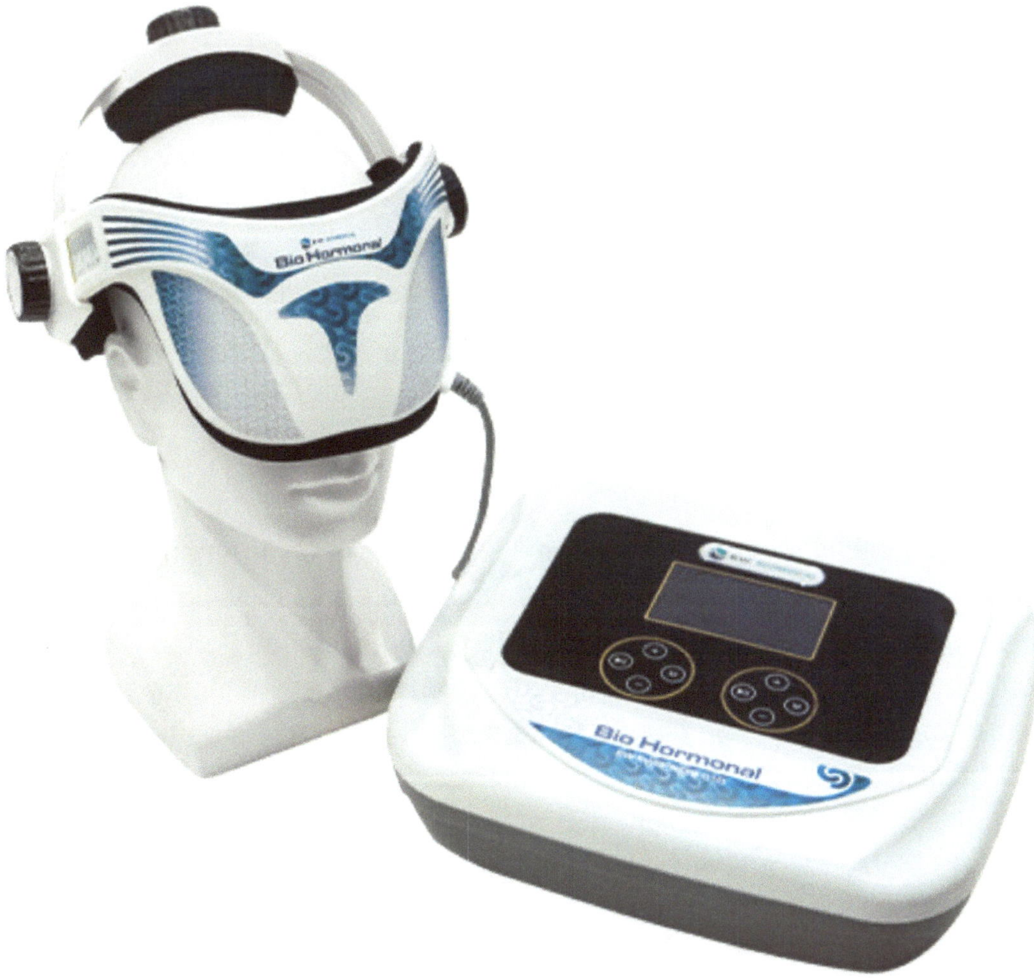

Source: European Wellness

Maintaining hormonal balance and facilitating the body's healing mechanisms have become paramount in a world increasingly shaped by modern lifestyles and environmental toxins. One innovative solution that combines these goals is the Bio Hormonal Modulator, a non-invasive pain reliever and healing accelerator that utilizes shortwave energy to stimulate blood flow, enhance glandular performance, and contribute to recovery. This versatile device can be employed both in clinical settings and at home, offering an effective approach to pain management and disease prevention.

A Non-Invasive Pain Reliever and Healing Accelerator

At the heart of the Bio Hormonal Modulator lies the use of shortwave energy, a cutting-edge technology that optimizes the body's natural restorative capabilities. By targeting the diencephalon and pituitary gland, this device stimulates the production of leukocytes, reinforcing the immune system's ability to combat diseases. This approach makes it a promising candidate for treating and preventing various health conditions.

Restoring Hormonal Balance

Hormonal imbalances often result from exposure to environmental toxins and unhealthy lifestyles, affecting our overall well-being and causing various health issues. The Bio Hormonal Modulator aims to rebalance these hormones by focusing on the pituitary gland, also known as the master gland, which governs the performance of other endocrine glands in the body. The device is particularly beneficial for those experiencing hormone-related disorders such as thyroid dysfunction, menstrual symptoms, depression, and anxiety. By optimizing hormonal function, the Bio Hormonal Modulator contributes to a more efficient recovery and helps manage the physical and emotional challenges that are often core in borderline disorders.

- **Improved Blood Circulation for Healing**. One of the device's key features is its ability to increase blood circulation, which is vital for healing. By facilitating better blood flow, the Bio Hormonal Modulator accelerates recovery and helps manage bodily pain effectively. It's a welcome relief for healthcare providers seeking non-invasive, drug-free solutions for their patients.

- **Efficiency and User-Friendly Operation**. The Bio Hormonal Modulator distinguishes itself with low power consumption. Generating a shortwave frequency of 27.12 MHz, the device operates on just 10 watts of electric energy. This energy-efficient approach saves on operating costs and reduces the environmental footprint. Furthermore, the device's easy operability ensures that professionals and non-professional users benefit from it. However, it's essential to note that individuals with metal implants, pacemakers, or foreign objects within their bodies should not use this device.

Versatile Applications for Brain Health and Hormonal Balance

The Bio Hormonal Modulator offers a wide range of health benefits, including:

1. Hormonal Balance: It addresses hormonally induced disorders such as thyroid dysfunction and menstrual symptoms, helping individuals regain their hormonal equilibrium.
2. Emotional Well-being: The device has been shown to alleviate symptoms of depression and anxiety, promoting mental health and overall quality of life.
3. Improved Sleep: For individuals with insomnia, the Bio Hormonal Modulator can provide relief, facilitating more restful sleep patterns.
4. Migraine Prevention: It can help prevent and ease migraines, reducing the frequency and severity of these painful episodes.
5. Neuroprotection: The device prevents brain cell loss and memory impairment, and maintains overall cognitive health.

The Bio Hormonal Modulator is a groundbreaking tool with the potential to revolutionize the recovery of borderline disorders and hormone-related health issues. Harnessing the power of shortwave energy offers non-invasive pain relief, accelerates healing, and contributes to overall well-being. As healthcare providers and individuals alike seek efficient and safe solutions, the Bio Hormonal Modulator stands out as a promising option for enhancing quality of life and promoting a healthier future.

Stress

Bio-hormonal modulators may assist in regulating endocrine pathways that become dysregulated during chronic stress. Persistent activation of the hypothalamic–pituitary–adrenal (HPA) axis can elevate cortisol levels, which may impair sleep patterns, cognitive flexibility, and emotional control. By influencing hormonal feedback loops, these modulators might help normalize stress-hormone fluctuations and support physiological relaxation responses.

Experimental models suggest that certain agents classified as bio-hormonal modulators can promote more adaptive autonomic balance, potentially lowering excessive sympathetic activation. This may support improvements in muscle tension, cardiovascular load, and digestive disturbances commonly associated with high stress states. Their use could also encourage parasympathetic activity, allowing enhanced physiological recovery after stress exposure.

Additionally, bio-hormonal modulation may help sustain neuroplastic processes linked to coping and resilience. More stable endocrine signaling may enhance communication between the prefrontal cortex and amygdala, potentially contributing to clearer emotional evaluation and more measured behavioral reactions to stressors.

Some modulators may also influence neuroimmune interactions associated with prolonged stress. By supporting a balanced inflammatory response, they could help preserve neuronal function in regions vulnerable to stress impacts such as the hippocampus. As a physiotherapeutic approach, these compounds can be incorporated into a broader plan aiming to maintain hormonal stability and functional stress responses, while promoting overall systemic homeostasis.

Anxiety

Bio-hormonal modulators may help reduce physiological hyperarousal that frequently accompanies anxiety-related disorders. Anxiety often involves heightened sensitivity to stress hormones such as adrenaline and cortisol. These modulators may help stabilize fluctuations in these hormones, potentially enabling individuals to maintain calmer bodily responses in uncertain or perceived threatening situations.

Research models show that improved hormonal balance may contribute to more regulated amygdala signaling. This could support a reduced tendency for alarm responses, enabling more proportional emotional interpretation of ambiguous stimuli. Neuroendocrine stabilization may also assist in diminishing anticipatory anxiety by moderating the body's preparatory "fight-or-flight" priming systems.

Some modulators are proposed to influence serotonin, GABA, and other neurotransmitters indirectly through hormone–brain communication pathways. This may support improvements in emotional control, muscle relaxation, and reduction of somatic tension contributing to anxiety symptoms such as rapid breathing or gastrointestinal discomfort.

Because anxiety often coexists with sleep disruption, supporting healthier circadian hormone rhythms could contribute to improved sleep quality and daytime stress tolerance. Physiology-guided modulation of endocrine activity may also enhance cognitive processing speed and attention, which anxiety often disrupts.

By supporting more adaptive endocrine-brain communication, bio-hormonal modulators may contribute to stabilization of physiological responses that underlie anxious states, offering potential value within comprehensive anxiety-management strategies.

Depression

Bio-hormonal modulators may assist in addressing endocrine disturbances linked to depressive symptoms. Depression can involve altered cortisol rhythms, reduced anabolic hormones, and impaired communication between endocrine signals and mood-regulating brain regions. By helping restore hormonal balance, these modulators might support improved motivation, sleep-wake cycles, and emotional stability.

Experimental evidence indicates that endocrine normalization may affect key neurotransmitter pathways. Stabilizing cortisol, thyroid-related signals, or sex-hormone activity may indirectly encourage serotonin and dopamine functioning, contributing to improved mood processing and reward sensitivity. These effects could help counteract anhedonia and reduced goal-directed behavior.

Chronic depression is sometimes associated with neuroinflammation and diminished hippocampal neurogenesis. Hormonal balance may support healthier neural environment and enhance plasticity in memory and cognitive control networks. This could be relevant for maintaining problem-solving skills, decision-making capacity, and learning-based emotional recovery.

Bio-hormonal modulators may also help improve energy regulation and reduce fatigue. Supporting more efficient hormone-driven metabolic processes might contribute to restored vitality and increased engagement in daily functioning.

Overall, integrating hormonal balance within physiotherapeutic approaches may offer a route to sustain emotional and cognitive functioning in individuals experiencing depressive symptoms, especially where stress physiology and neuroendocrine pathways are prominently involved.

Morphogenetic Harmonizer System, Scalar Plasma Wave Modulator

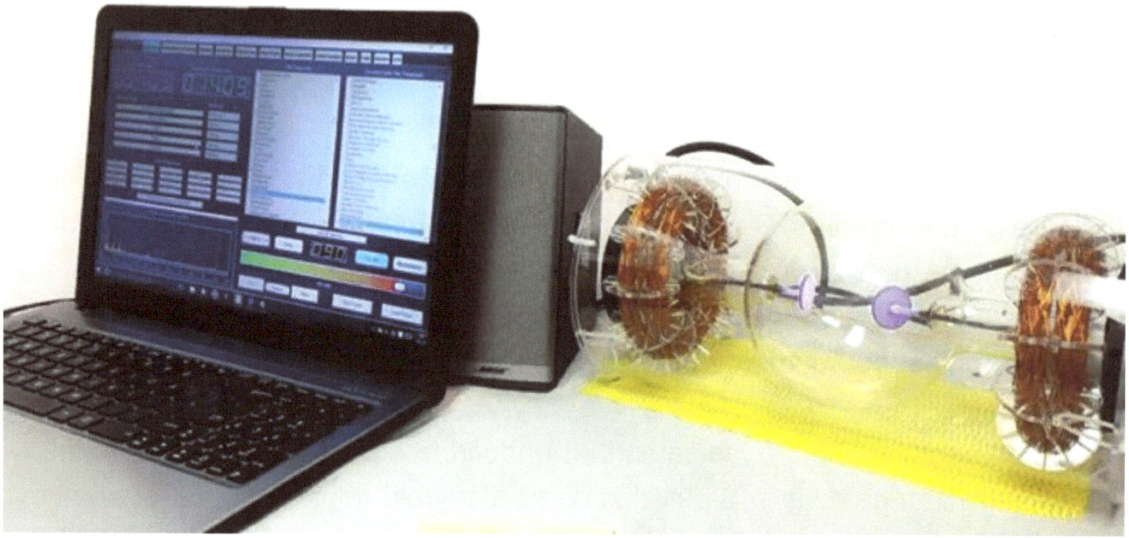

Source: European Wellness

The Scalar Plasma Wave Modulator represents a multifaceted approach to health and well-being, claiming to harmonise critical systems within the body, particularly the immune and cellular regenerative systems. It also proposes to address the reprogramming of introns (often referred to as junk DNA) to reverse mutations within these regions. Let's delve deeper into the concepts and mechanisms associated with the Scalar Plasma Wave Modulator.

Harmonisation of Immune System and Cellular Regenerative System:

The Scalar Plasma Wave Modulator is designed to harmonise two fundamental systems in the body simultaneously:

Immune System: The immune system is responsible for identifying and combating foreign invaders, such as pathogens and abnormal cells. While it plays a vital role in protecting the body, it may not directly contribute to the regeneration of damaged cells.

Cellular Regenerative System: This lesser-known system is considered electromagnetic in nature and relies on longitudinal scalar waves. As proposed by the late Dr. Robert Becker, these waves could have a role in the regeneration and repair of damaged cells and tissues. The Scalar Plasma Wave Modulator aims to optimise the function of both systems, promoting overall health and healing.

- **Reprogramming Introns (Junk DNA):** One of the claims associated with this modulator is the reprogramming of introns, often referred to as junk DNA. Introns are regions within the DNA that do not encode proteins, and their exact function is still an area of scientific investigation. The device suggests reprograming these introns by altering the morphogenetic encryption lattice, potentially reversing mutations or promoting beneficial changes within these non-coding regions.
- **Creation of Multidimensional Scalar Energy Fields:** The Scalar Plasma Wave Modulator is described as capable of creating multidimensional scalar magnetic energy fields. These fields can extend up to twelve to twenty-four feet away from the device. Such fields are believed

to encompass deliberately constructed, enfolded components, including phase conjugate waves.

- **Primary Electrical Conductivity Pathway:** The device proposes that the primary electrical conductivity pathway within the cellular regenerative system is not through the electron shells of atoms but instead involves nuclei-to-nuclei scalar electromagnetic "biopotential levels." This implies that the scalar energy pathway plays a significant role in the cellular regenerative process.
- **BioRegenesis Technologies:** BioRegenesis technologies, as a broader concept, encompass scalar mechanics that leverage scalar waves' natural power to influence the body's morphogenetic field manifestation blueprint. These technologies incorporate various elements:
    - Light (Color): Color is used as a scalar wave technology to influence the morphogenetic field.
    - Symbols: Symbols, often associated with eternality and base-12 geomancy, are utilised to create specific scalar wave blueprints.
    - Sound: Sound, when harnessed in specific arrays of inner light and magnetic energy, is projected into the morphogenetic field, influencing it at an energetic level.

  Geomancy, in this context, refers to the arrangement of light and sound within the morphogenetic field blueprint. This arrangement is constructed based on specific sound frequencies infused with transharmonic electrical flux.
- **Language and Scalar Templates:** The Scalar Plasma Wave Modulator suggests that written and spoken languages embody fragments of sound vibration scalar templates found in the body's morphogenetic field manifestation blueprint. Written language symbols are viewed as scalar standing wave instructions that translate into sound vibration electrical impulses within the body's scalar field template. These electrical impulses are believed to affect the introns, the physical body, and consciousness itself.

In essence, the Scalar Plasma Wave Modulator proposes a complex interplay of scalar energy, colour, symbols, and sound to influence the body's morphogenetic field, potentially impacting the immune system, cellular regeneration, and the reprogramming of introns. The Morphogenetic Harmonizer System - Scalar Plasma Wave Modulator is an innovative device with the potential to influence borderline disorders management by addressing the autonomic nervous system, stress reduction, and cellular detoxification. These technologies operate based on principles related to scalar waves and electromagnetic energy fields. Although they are not conventional medical treatments, they are sometimes explored as complementary approaches in the realm of holistic and alternative medicine.

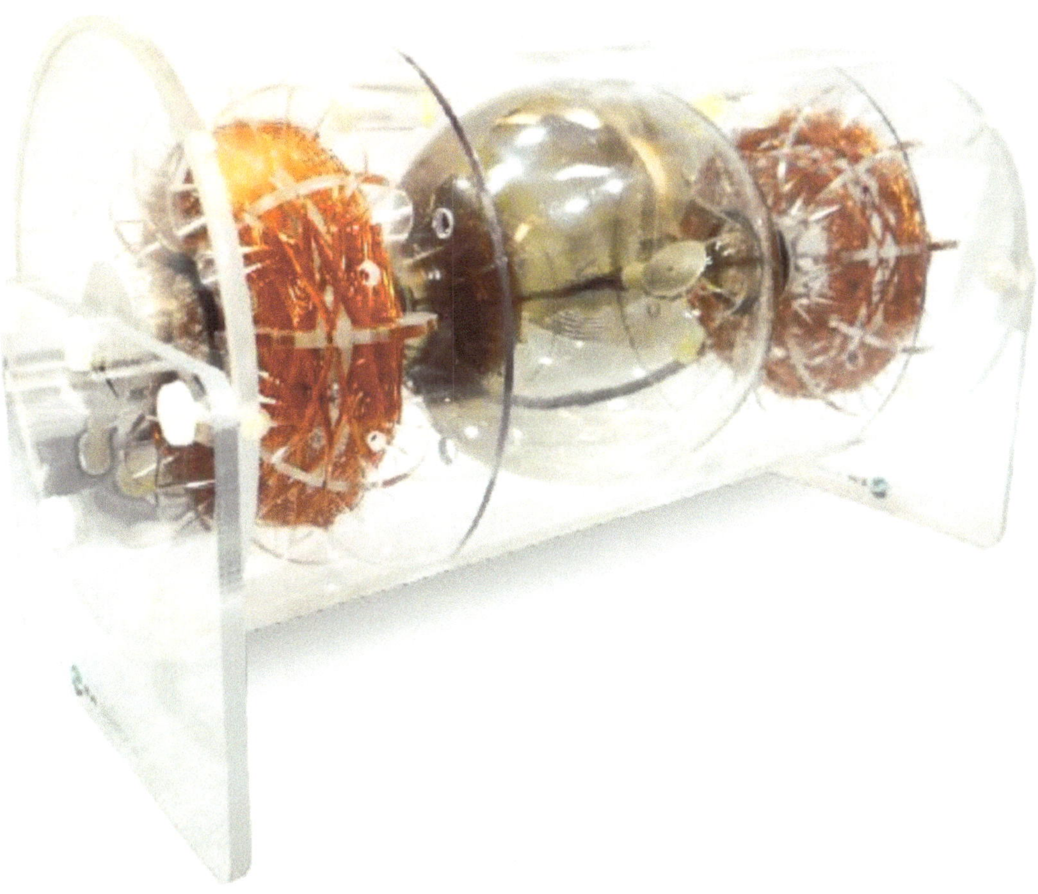

Source: European Wellness.

The Morphogenetic Harmonizer System protects, enhances, and harmonizes the autonomic nervous system. It aims to achieve these effects by:

- Relieving Stressors: Stress can have detrimental effects on health, and its management is crucial in the recovery of borderline disorders. The system may help individuals reduce stress levels through relaxation techniques and energy balancing.
- Transmuting Negative Habitual Patterns: Addressing negative habitual patterns of thought and behaviour can be essential for overall well-being and recovery. The system may help identify and transform such patterns.
- Supporting Relaxation: Relaxation is vital for patients with borderline disorders, as it can aid in reducing tension and promoting a healing environment.
- Cellular Detoxification: Detoxification processes can play a role in recovering from borderline disorders-related damage. Cellular detoxification is believed to aid in eliminating harmful substances from the body.
- Healing from Stress: Stress can hinder the body's healing processes. The system may indirectly support the body's natural healing mechanisms by relieving stressors and promoting relaxation.
- Autonomic Nervous System Balancing: Balancing the autonomic nervous system can contribute to overall health and well-being. It may help regulate processes like heart rate, blood pressure, and stress response.

Harmonizing Electromagnetic Fields: Scalar waves and electromagnetic fields are believed to have an impact on the body's subtle energy systems. Harmonizing these fields could theoretically promote a state of balance and harmony.

Bibliography

Admiraal, W. M., & Huisman, S. D. (2013). Current and future applications of stem cells in neurodegenerative diseases. *Advances in Stem Cells*, *2013*, Article ID 708529.

Anacker, C., & Hen, R. (2017). Adult hippocampal neurogenesis and cognitive flexibility—linking memory and mood. *Nature Reviews Neuroscience*, *18*(6), 335-346.

Anacker, C., Zunszain, P. A., Cattaneo, A., Carvalho, L. A., Garabedian, M. J., Thuret, S., ... & Pariante, C. M. (2011). Antidepressants increase human hippocampal neurogenesis by activating the glucocorticoid receptor. *Molecular Psychiatry*, *16*(7), 738-750.

Arnsten, A. F. (2009). Stress signalling pathways that impair prefrontal cortex structure and function. *Nature Reviews Neuroscience*, *10*(6), 410-422.

Autry, A. E., & Monteggia, L. M. (2012). Brain-derived neurotrophic factor and neuropsychiatric disorders. *Pharmacological Reviews*, *64*(2), 238-258.

Berlim, M. T., Van den Eynde, F., Tovar-Perdomo, S., & Daskalakis, Z. J. (2014). Response, remission and drop-out rates following high-frequency repetitive transcranial magnetic stimulation (rTMS) for treating major depression: a systematic review and meta-analysis of randomized, double-blind and sham-controlled trials. *Psychological Medicine*, *44*(2), 225-239.

Boku, S., Nakagawa, S., Takamura, N., Kato, A., Takebayashi, M., Hisaoka-Nakashima, K., ... & Kusumi, I. (2018). Neural stem cells for the treatment of psychiatric disorders: Current status and future direction. *Psychiatry and Clinical Neurosciences*, *72*(12), 899-908.

Boldrini, M., Fulmore, C. A., Tartt, A. N., Simeon, L. R., Pavlova, I., Poposka, V., ... & Mann, J. J. (2018). Human hippocampal neurogenesis persists throughout aging. *Cell Stem Cell*, *22*(4), 589-599.

Bremner, J. D. (2006). Traumatic stress: effects on the brain. *Dialogues in Clinical Neuroscience*, *8*(4), 445-461.

Bromet, E., Andrade, L. H., Hwang, I., Sampson, N. A., Alonso, J., De Girolamo, G., ... & Kessler, R. C. (2011). Cross-national epidemiology of DSM-IV major depressive episode. *BMC Medicine*, *9*(1), 1-16.

Brunoni, A. R., Moffa, A. H., Fregni, F., Palm, U., Padberg, F., Blumberger, D. M., ... & Loo, C. K. (2016). Transcranial direct current stimulation for acute major depressive episodes: meta-analysis of individual patient data. *British Journal of Psychiatry*, *208*(6), 522-531.

Camfield, D. A., Sarris, J., & Berk, M. (2011). Nutraceuticals in the treatment of obsessive compulsive disorder (OCD): a review of mechanistic and clinical evidence. *Progress in Neuro-Psychopharmacology and Biological Psychiatry*, *35*(4), 887-895.

Carpenter, L. L., Janicak, P. G., Aaronson, S. T., Boyadjis, T., Brock, D. G., Cook, I. A., ... & Demitrack, M. A. (2012). Transcranial magnetic stimulation (TMS) for major depression: a multisite, naturalistic, observational study of acute treatment outcomes in clinical practice. *Depression and Anxiety*, *29*(7), 587-596.

Castrén, E., & Rantamäki, T. (2010). The role of BDNF and its receptors in depression and antidepressant drug action: reactivation of developmental plasticity. *Developmental Neurobiology*, *70*(5), 289-297.

Chrousos, G. P. (2009). Stress and disorders of the stress system. *Nature Reviews Endocrinology*, *5*(7), 374-381.

Czeisler, M. É., Lane, R. I., Petrosky, E., Wiley, J. F., Christensen, A., Njai, R., ... & Rajaratnam, S. M. (2020). Mental health, substance use, and suicidal ideation during the COVID-19 pandemic. *Morbidity and Mortality Weekly Report*, *69*(32), 1049-1057.

Dantzer, R., O'Connor, J. C., Freund, G. G., Johnson, R. W., & Kelley, K. W. (2008). From inflammation to sickness and depression: when the immune system subjugates the brain. *Nature Reviews Neuroscience*, *9*(1), 46-56.

De Kloet, E. R., Joëls, M., & Holsboer, F. (2005). Stress and the brain: from adaptation to disease. *Nature Reviews Neuroscience*, *6*(6), 463-475.

Deng, Z. D., Lisanby, S. H., & Peterchev, A. V. (2013). Electric field depth–focality tradeoff in transcranial magnetic stimulation: simulation comparison of 50 coil designs. *Brain Stimulation*, *6*(1), 1-13.

Drevets, W. C., Price, J. L., & Furey, M. L. (2008). Brain structural and functional abnormalities in mood disorders: implications for neurocircuitry models of depression. *Brain Structure and Function*, *213*(1-2), 93-118.

Drevets, W. C., Savitz, J., & Trimble, M. (2008). The subgenual anterior cingulate cortex in mood disorders. *CNS Spectrums*, *13*(8), 663-681.

Duman, R. S., & Aghajanian, G. K. (2012). Synaptic dysfunction in depression: potential therapeutic targets. *Science*, *338*(6103), 68-72.

Duman, R. S., & Monteggia, L. M. (2006). A neurotrophic model for stress-related mood disorders. *Biological Psychiatry*, *59*(12), 1116-1127.

Duman, R. S., Heninger, G. R., & Nestler, E. J. (1997). A molecular and cellular theory of depression. *Archives of General Psychiatry*, *54*(7), 597-606.

Duman, R. S., Malberg, J., & Nakagawa, S. (2001). Regulation of adult neurogenesis by psychotropic drugs and stress. *Journal of Pharmacology and Experimental Therapeutics*, *299*(2), 401-407.

Dwivedi, Y. (2009). Brain-derived neurotrophic factor: role in depression and suicide. *Neuropsychiatric Disease and Treatment*, *5*, 433-449.

Eisch, A. J., & Petrik, D. (2012). Depression and hippocampal neurogenesis: a road to remission? *Science*, *338*(6103), 72-75.

Elkins, G., Johnson, A., & Fisher, W. (2012). Cognitive hypnotherapy for pain management. *American Journal of Clinical Hypnosis*, *54*(4), 294-310.

Eroglu, D., Akar, H., Eker, S. S., & Ozturk, M. (2020). Potential therapeutic role of ozone therapy in neurological diseases: a review. *Medical Gas Research*, *10*(1), 38-43.

Etkin, A., & Wager, T. D. (2007). Functional neuroimaging of anxiety: a meta-analysis of emotional processing in PTSD, social anxiety disorder, and specific phobia. *American Journal of Psychiatry*, *164*(10), 1476-1488.

Falk, A., & Jönsson, M. E. (2019). Human pluripotent stem cells in psychiatric research. *Neuropsychopharmacology*, *44*(1), 245-246.

Felger, J. C., & Lotrich, F. E. (2013). Inflammatory cytokines in depression: neurobiological mechanisms and therapeutic implications. *Neuroscience*, *246*, 199-229.

Felitti, V. J., Anda, R. F., Nordenberg, D., Williamson, D. F., Spitz, A. M., Edwards, V., ... & Marks, J. S. (1998). Relationship of childhood abuse and household dysfunction to many of the leading causes of death in adults. *American Journal of Preventive Medicine*, *14*(4), 245-258.

Ferrari, A. J., Charlson, F. J., Norman, R. E., Patten, S. B., Freedman, G., Murray, C. J., ... & Whiteford, H. A. (2013). Burden of depressive disorders by country, sex, age, and year: findings from the global burden of disease study 2010. *PLoS Medicine*, *10*(11), e1001547.

Frodl, T., & O'Keane, V. (2013). How does the brain deal with cumulative stress? A review with focus on developmental stress, HPA axis function and hippocampal structure in humans. *Neurobiology of Disease*, *52*, 24-37.

Gage, F. H., & Temple, S. (2013). Neural stem cells: generating and regenerating the brain. *Neuron*, *80*(3), 588-601.

George, M. S., Lisanby, S. H., Avery, D., McDonald, W. M., Durkalski, V., Pavlicova, M., ... & Sackeim, H. A. (2010). Daily left prefrontal transcranial magnetic stimulation therapy for major depressive disorder: a sham-controlled randomized trial. *Archives of General Psychiatry*, *67*(5), 507-516.

Geracioti Jr, T. D., & Orth, D. N. (2018). CRF and vasopressin infusions as probe tests in depression and anxiety. *Psychopharmacology Bulletin*, *28*(3), 349-352.

Griebel, G., & Holsboer, F. (2012). Neuropeptide receptor ligands as drugs for psychiatric diseases: the end of the beginning? *Nature Reviews Drug Discovery*, *11*(6), 462-478.

Hadanny, A., & Efrati, S. (2020). The hyperoxic-hypoxic paradox. *Biomolecules*, *10*(6), 958.

Hadanny, A., Abbott, S., Suzin, G., Bechor, Y., & Efrati, S. (2018). Effect of hyperbaric oxygen therapy on chronic neurocognitive deficits of post-traumatic brain injury patients: retrospective analysis. *BMJ Open*, *8*(9), e023387.

Hamilton, J. P., Etkin, A., Furman, D. J., Lemus, M. G., Johnson, R. F., & Gotlib, I. H. (2012). Functional neuroimaging of major depressive disorder: a meta-analysis and new integration of baseline activation and neural response data. *American Journal of Psychiatry*, *169*(7), 693-703.

Hasin, D. S., Sarvet, A. L., Meyers, J. L., Saha, T. D., Ruan, W. J., Stohl, M., & Grant, B. F. (2018). Epidemiology of adult DSM-5 major depressive disorder and its specifiers in the United States. *JAMA Psychiatry*, *75*(4), 336-346.

Hashimoto, K., Shimizu, E., & Iyo, M. (2004). Critical role of brain-derived neurotrophic factor in mood disorders. *Brain Research Reviews*, *45*(2), 104-114.

Herman, J. P., McKlveen, J. M., Ghosal, S., Kopp, B., Wulsin, A., Makinson, R., ... & Myers, B. (2016). Regulation of the hypothalamic-pituitary-adrenocortical stress response. *Comprehensive Physiology*, *6*(2), 603-621.

Hill, A. S., Sahay, A., & Hen, R. (2015). Increasing adult hippocampal neurogenesis is sufficient to reduce anxiety and depression-like behaviors. *Neuropsychopharmacology*, *40*(10), 2368-2378.

Holmes, A., Heilig, M., Rupniak, N. M., Steckler, T., & Griebel, G. (2003). Neuropeptide systems as novel therapeutic targets for depression and anxiety disorders. *Trends in Pharmacological Sciences*, *24*(11), 580-588.

Holtzheimer, P. E., & Mayberg, H. S. (2011). Deep brain stimulation for psychiatric disorders. *Annual Review of Neuroscience*, *34*, 289-307.

Huang, L., & Obenaus, A. (2011). Hyperbaric oxygen therapy for traumatic brain injury. *Medical Gas Research*, *1*(1), 1-13.

Jin, K., Xie, L., Childs, J., Sun, Y., Mao, X. O., Logvinova, A., & Greenberg, D. A. (2003). Cerebral neurogenesis is induced by intranasal administration of growth factors. *Annals of Neurology*, *53*(3), 405-409.

Juruena, M. F., Bocharova, M., Agustini, B., & Young, A. H. (2018). Atypical depression and non-atypical depression: Is HPA axis function a biomarker? A systematic review. *Journal of Affective Disorders*, *233*, 45-67.

Kastin, A. J., & Akerstrom, V. (1999). Orexin A but not orexin B rapidly enters brain from blood by simple diffusion. *Journal of Pharmacology and Experimental Therapeutics*, *289*(1), 219-223.

Kempermann, G., Song, H., & Gage, F. H. (2015). Neurogenesis in the adult hippocampus. *Cold Spring Harbor Perspectives in Biology*, *7*(9), a018812.

Kessler, R. C., Berglund, P., Demler, O., Jin, R., Merikangas, K. R., & Walters, E. E. (2005). Lifetime prevalence and age-of-onset distributions of DSM-IV disorders in the National Comorbidity Survey Replication. *Archives of General Psychiatry*, *62*(6), 593-602.

Kessler, R. C., Chiu, W. T., Demler, O., & Walters, E. E. (2005). Prevalence, severity, and comorbidity of 12-month DSM-IV disorders in the National Comorbidity Survey Replication. *Archives of General Psychiatry*, *62*(6), 617-627.

Khandaker, G. M., Pearson, R. M., Zammit, S., Lewis, G., & Jones, P. B. (2014). Association of serum interleukin 6 and C-reactive protein in childhood with depression and psychosis in young adult life. *JAMA Psychiatry*, *71*(10), 1121-1128.

Köhler, C. A., Freitas, T. H., Maes, M., de Andrade, N. Q., Liu, C. S., Fernandes, B. S., ... & Carvalho, A. F. (2017). Peripheral cytokine and chemokine alterations in depression: a meta-analysis of 82 studies. *Acta Psychiatrica Scandinavica*, *135*(5), 373-387.

Krishnan, V., & Nestler, E. J. (2008). The molecular neurobiology of depression. *Nature*, *455*(7215), 894-902.

Lefaucheur, J. P., André-Obadia, N., Antal, A., Ayache, S. S., Baeken, C., Benninger, D. H., ... & Garcia-Larrea, L. (2014). Evidence-based guidelines on the therapeutic use of repetitive transcranial magnetic stimulation (rTMS). *Clinical Neurophysiology*, *125*(11), 2150-2206.

Levy, M. J., Boulle, F., Steinbusch, H. W., van den Hove, D. L., Kenis, G., & Lanfumey, L. (2018). Neurotrophic factors and neuroplasticity pathways in the pathophysiology and treatment of depression. *Psychopharmacology*, *235*(8), 2195-2220.

Lucassen, P. J., Meerlo, P., Naylor, A. S., Van Dam, A. M., Dayer, A. G., Fuchs, E., ... & Czéh, B. (2010). Regulation of adult neurogenesis by stress, sleep disruption, exercise and inflammation: Implications for depression and antidepressant action. *European Neuropsychopharmacology*, *20*(1), 1-17.

Luo, J., Daniels, S. B., Lennington, J. B., Notti, R. Q., & Conover, J. C. (2006). The aging neurogenic subventricular zone. *Aging Cell*, *5*(2), 139-152.

Lupien, S. J., McEwen, B. S., Gunnar, M. R., & Heim, C. (2009). Effects of stress throughout the lifespan on the brain, behaviour and cognition. *Nature Reviews Neuroscience*, *10*(6), 434-445.

Maeng, S., & Zarate Jr, C. A. (2007). The role of glutamate in mood disorders: results from the ketamine in major depression study and the presumed cellular mechanism underlying its antidepressant effects. *Current Psychiatry Reports*, *9*(6), 467-474.

Maes, M., Yirmyia, R., Noraberg, J., Brene, S., Hibbeln, J., Perini, G., ... & Maj, M. (2009). The inflammatory & neurodegenerative (I&ND) hypothesis of depression:

leads for future research and new drug developments in depression. *Metabolic Brain Disease*, *24*(1), 27-53.

Malberg, J. E., Eisch, A. J., Nestler, E. J., & Duman, R. S. (2000). Chronic antidepressant treatment increases neurogenesis in adult rat hippocampus. *Journal of Neuroscience*, *20*(24), 9104-9110.

Marlatt, M. W., Lucassen, P. J., & van Praag, H. (2010). Comparison of neurogenic effects of fluoxetine, duloxetine and running in mice. *Brain Research*, *1341*, 93-99.

Martinowich, K., Manji, H., & Lu, B. (2007). New insights into BDNF function in depression and anxiety. *Nature Neuroscience*, *10*(9), 1089-1093.

Mathé, A. A., Jiménez-Vasquez, P. A., Theodorsson, E., & Lindström, L. H. (2015). Neuropeptides in neuropsychiatric disorders: neuropeptide Y and corticotropin-releasing hormone in depression and anxiety. *Progress in Molecular Biology and Translational Science*, *136*, 323-346.

Mayberg, H. S. (2009). Targeted electrode-based modulation of neural circuits for depression. *Journal of Clinical Investigation*, *119*(4), 717-725.

McEwen, B. S. (2007). Physiology and neurobiology of stress and adaptation: central role of the brain. *Physiological Reviews*, *87*(3), 873-904.

McEwen, B. S., & Gianaros, P. J. (2011). Stress-and allostasis-induced brain plasticity. *Annual Review of Medicine*, *62*, 431-445.

McLaughlin, K. A., Conron, K. J., Koenen, K. C., & Gilman, S. E. (2010). Childhood adversity, adult stressful life events, and risk of past-year psychiatric disorder: a test of the stress sensitization hypothesis. *Psychological Medicine*, *40*(10), 1647-1658.

Miller, A. H., & Raison, C. L. (2016). The role of inflammation in depression: from evolutionary imperative to modern treatment target. *Nature Reviews Immunology*, *16*(1), 22-34.

Miller, A. H., Maletic, V., & Raison, C. L. (2009). Inflammation and its discontents: the role of cytokines in the pathophysiology of major depression. *Biological Psychiatry*, *65*(9), 732-741.

Moffitt, T. E., Caspi, A., Taylor, A., Kokaua, J., Milne, B. J., Polanczyk, G., & Poulton, R. (2010). How common are common mental disorders? Evidence that lifetime prevalence rates are doubled by prospective versus retrospective ascertainment. *Psychological Medicine*, *40*(6), 899-909.

Myczkowski, M. L., Fernandes, A., Moreno, M., Valiengo, L., Lafer, B., Moreno, R. A., ... & Brunoni, A. R. (2018). Cognitive outcomes of TMS treatment in bipolar depression: safety data from a randomized controlled trial. *Journal of Affective Disorders*, *235*, 20-26.

Nestler, E. J., Barrot, M., DiLeone, R. J., Eisch, A. J., Gold, S. J., & Monteggia, L. M. (2002). Neurobiology of depression. *Neuron*, *34*(1), 13-25.

Neumann, I. D., & Landgraf, R. (2012). Balance of brain oxytocin and vasopressin: implications for anxiety, depression, and social behaviors. *Trends in Neurosciences*, *35*(11), 649-659.

Pariante, C. M., & Lightman, S. L. (2008). The HPA axis in major depression: classical theories and new developments. *Trends in Neurosciences*, *31*(9), 464-468.

Perera, T., George, M. S., Grammer, G., Janicak, P. G., Pascual-Leone, A., & Wirecki, T. S. (2016). The clinical TMS society consensus review and treatment recommendations for TMS therapy for major depressive disorder. *Brain Stimulation*, *9*(3), 336-346.

Phelps, E. A., & LeDoux, J. E. (2005). Contributions of the amygdala to emotion processing: from animal models to human behavior. *Neuron*, *48*(2), 175-187.

Pittenger, C., & Duman, R. S. (2008). Stress, depression, and neuroplasticity: a convergence of mechanisms. *Neuropsychopharmacology*, *33*(1), 88-109.

Popoli, M., Yan, Z., McEwen, B. S., & Sanacora, G. (2012). The stressed synapse: the impact of stress and glucocorticoids on glutamate transmission. *Nature Reviews Neuroscience*, *13*(1), 22-37.

Price, J. L., & Drevets, W. C. (2012). Neural circuits underlying the pathophysiology of mood disorders. *Trends in Cognitive Sciences*, *16*(1), 61-71.

Raichle, M. E. (2015). The brain's default mode network. *Annual Review of Neuroscience*, *38*, 433-447.

Raison, C. L., Capuron, L., & Miller, A. H. (2006). Cytokines sing the blues: inflammation and the pathogenesis of depression. *Trends in Immunology*, *27*(1), 24-31.

Rajkowska, G., & Miguel-Hidalgo, J. J. (2007). Gliogenesis and glial pathology in depression. *CNS & Neurological Disorders-Drug Targets*, *6*(3), 219-233.

Re, L., Martínez-Sánchez, G., Bordicchia, M., Malcangi, G., Pocognoli, A., Morales-Segura, M. A., ... & Fernández-Montequín, J. I. (2008). Is ozone pre-conditioning effect linked to Nrf2/EpRE activation pathway in vivo? A preliminary result. *European Journal of Pharmacology*, *590*(1-3), 158-161.

Ressler, K. J., & Mayberg, H. S. (2007). Targeting abnormal neural circuits in mood and anxiety disorders: from the laboratory to the clinic. *Nature Neuroscience*, *10*(9), 1116-1124.

Ressler, K. J., & Nemeroff, C. B. (2000). Role of serotonergic and noradrenergic systems in the pathophysiology of depression and anxiety disorders. *Depression and Anxiety*, *12*(S1), 2-19.

Russo, S. J., & Nestler, E. J. (2013). The brain reward circuitry in mood disorders. *Nature Reviews Neuroscience*, *14*(9), 609-625.

Sahay, A., & Hen, R. (2007). Adult hippocampal neurogenesis in depression. *Nature Neuroscience*, *10*(9), 1110-1115.

Salehpour, F., Mahmoudi, J., Kamari, F., Sadigh-Eteghad, S., Rasta, S. H., & Hamblin, M. R. (2018). Brain photobiomodulation therapy: a narrative review. *Molecular Neurobiology*, *55*(8), 6601-6636.

Sanacora, G., Treccani, G., & Popoli, M. (2012). Towards a glutamate hypothesis of depression: an emerging frontier of neuropsychopharmacology for mood disorders. *Neuropharmacology*, *62*(1), 63-77.

Sapolsky, R. M. (2015). Stress and the brain: individual variability and the inverted-U. *Nature Neuroscience*, *18*(10), 1344-1346.

Setiawan, E., Wilson, A. A., Mizrahi, R., Rusjan, P. M., Miler, L., Rajkowska, G., ... & Meyer, J. H. (2015). Role of translocator protein density, a marker of neuroinflammation, in the brain during major depressive episodes. *JAMA Psychiatry*, *72*(3), 268-275.

Shin, L. M., & Liberzon, I. (2010). The neurocircuitry of fear, stress, and anxiety disorders. *Neuropsychopharmacology*, *35*(1), 169-191.

Shin, L. M., Rauch, S. L., & Pitman, R. K. (2006). Amygdala, medial prefrontal cortex, and hippocampal function in PTSD. *Annals of the New York Academy of Sciences*, *1071*(1), 67-79.

Small, D. M., Zatorre, R. J., Dagher, A., Evans, A. C., & Jones-Gotman, M. (2001). Changes in brain activity related to eating chocolate. *Brain*, *124*(9), 1720-1733.

Snyder, J. S., Soumier, A., Brewer, M., Pickel, J., & Cameron, H. A. (2011). Adult hippocampal neurogenesis buffers stress responses and depressive behaviour. *Nature*, *476*(7361), 458-461.

Stockmeier, C. A., Mahajan, G. J., Konick, L. C., Overholser, J. C., Jurjus, G. J., Meltzer, H. Y., ... & Rajkowska, G. (2004). Cellular changes in the postmortem hippocampus in major depression. *Biological Psychiatry*, *56*(9), 640-650.

Substance Abuse and Mental Health Services Administration. (2020). *Key substance use and mental health indicators in the United States: Results from the 2019 National Survey on Drug Use and Health* (HHS Publication No. PEP20-07-01-001, NSDUH Series H-55). Rockville, MD: Center for Behavioral Health Statistics and Quality.

Tfilin, M., & Turgeman, G. (2019). Interrelationship between adult neurogenesis and Alzheimer's disease: A new therapeutic approach? *Journal of Alzheimer's Disease*, *67*(4), 1073-1087.

Toda, T., Parylak, S. L., Linker, S. B., & Gage, F. H. (2019). The role of adult hippocampal neurogenesis in brain health and disease. *Molecular Psychiatry*, *24*(1), 67-87.

Twenge, J. M., Cooper, A. B., Joiner, T. E., Duffy, M. E., & Binau, S. G. (2019). Age, period, and cohort trends in mood disorder indicators and suicide-related outcomes in a nationally representative dataset, 2005–2017. *Journal of Abnormal Psychology*, *128*(3), 185-199.

Ulrich-Lai, Y. M., & Herman, J. P. (2009). Neural regulation of endocrine and autonomic stress responses. *Nature Reviews Neuroscience*, *10*(6), 397-409.

Winner, B., & Winkler, J. (2015). Adult neurogenesis in neurodegenerative diseases. *Cold Spring Harbor Perspectives in Biology*, *7*(4), a021287.

Young, E. A., Abelson, J. L., & Cameron, O. G. (2004). Effect of comorbid anxiety disorders on the hypothalamic-pituitary-adrenal axis response to a social stressor in major depression. *Biological Psychiatry*, *56*(2), 113-120.

Zhao, C., Deng, W., & Gage, F. H. (2008). Mechanisms and functional implications of adult neurogenesis. *Cell*, *132*(4), 645-660.

Zorrilla, E. P., & Koob, G. F. (2019). Progress in corticotropin-releasing factor-1 antagonist development. *Drug Discovery Today*, *24*(2), 366-382.

www.ingramcontent.com/pod-product-compliance
Lightning Source LLC
LaVergne TN
LVHW070343240926
848802LV00003B/7